TWINKIE, DECONSTRUCTED

STEVE ETTLINGER has been an author, editor, and book producer since 1985, and has created over a dozen popular reference books that have sold over a million copies. He has appeared on *The Today Show*, *CBS This Morning*, *Good Morning America*, *The Montel Williams Show*, CNN, Fox News, *Live with Regis and Kathie Lee*, *Nightline*, NPR's *The Leonard Lopate Show*, the Food Network, and dozens of other television and radio shows and networks.

Ettlinger lived in Paris for six years, where he managed to eat at many of the world's finest restaurants. He has previously worked as an assistant chef and enjoys old home repair and renovation, cooking, sailing, and African drumming. A graduate of Tufts University, he lives in New York City with his wife, Gusty Lange, and their two children.

"A delightful romp through the food processing industry."

—*Publishers Weekly*

"If you want to explore all the unpronounceable and highly suspect ingredients we consume daily, what better starting point could you choose than that classic, golden, crème-filled cake reputedly capable of withstanding a nuclear holocaust?"   —*The Washington Post Book World*

"An insightful look into the processed food industry."   —*Library Journal*

"This fantastical, bionic journey is chronicled ingredient-by-ingredient in Steve Ettlinger's thorough and often charming [book]." —NYCnosh.com

"Ettlinger digs deep and does it skillfully."   —*The Denver Post*

"Slim, bearded, and armed with a streak of geeky good humor, Ettlinger is like a professor with a passion for food. When he orders a hot chocolate with whipped cream from Starbucks 'for research purposes,' he's telling the truth."   —*New York Daily News*

"Ettlinger shares his enriched and tasty Twinkie tale one morsel at a time. The effect is satiating."   —boldtype.com

Twinkie,
Deconstructed

My Journey to Discover How the
Ingredients Found in Processed Foods
Are Grown, Mined (Yes, Mined), and
Manipulated into What America Eats

Steve Ettlinger

A PLUME BOOK

PLUME
Published by the Penguin Group
Penguin Group (USA) Inc., 375 Hudson Street, New York, New York 10014, U.S.A. •
Penguin Group (Canada), 90 Eglinton Avenue East, Suite 700, Toronto, Ontario, Canada
M4P 2Y3 (a division of Pearson Penguin Canada Inc.) • Penguin Books Ltd., 80 Strand,
London WC2R 0RL, England • Penguin Ireland, 25 St. Stephen's Green, Dublin 2, Ire-
land (a division of Penguin Books Ltd.) • Penguin Group (Australia), 250 Camberwell
Road, Camberwell, Victoria 3124, Australia (a division of Pearson Australia Group Pty.
Ltd.) • Penguin Books India Pvt. Ltd., 11 Community Centre, Panchsheel Park, New
Delhi – 110 017, India • Penguin Group (NZ), 67 Apollo Drive, Rosedale, North Shore
0632, New Zealand (a division of Pearson New Zealand Ltd.) • Penguin Books (South
Africa) (Pty.) Ltd., 24 Sturdee Avenue, Rosebank, Johannesburg 2196, South Africa

Penguin Books Ltd., Registered Offices: 80 Strand, London WC2R 0RL, England

Published by Plume, a member of Penguin Group (USA) Inc. Previously published in a
Hudson Street Press edition.

First Plume Printing, March 2008

10 9 8 7 6 5 4 3 2

Ⓟ REGISTERED TRADEMARK—MARCA REGISTRADA

The Library of Congress has catalogued the Hudson Street Press edition as follows:
Ettlinger, Steve.
  Twinkie, deconstructed : my journey to discover how the ingredients found in pro-
cessed foods are grown, mined (yes, mined), and manipulated into what America eats. /
Steve Eittlinger.
     p. cm.
  ISBN 978-1-59463-018-7 (hc.)
  ISBN 978-0-452-28928-4 (pbk.)
  1. Food additives.   2. Processed foods.   3. Twinkies (Trademark)   I. Title.
TX553.A3E85 2007
641.3'08—dc22   2006030013

Printed in the United States of America
Original hardcover design by Eve L. Kirch

To Dylan and Chelsea
and
To those of us who have spent many a dull
moment staring, uncomprehending, at the
ingredient list on the label of some packaged
food (you have plenty of company).
Now you can read this book instead.

Tell me what you eat,
and I will tell you what you are.

—Jean Anthelme Brillat-Savarin
The Physiology of Taste

ACKNOWLEDGMENTS

First and foremost, I'm grateful to my children, Chelsea and Dylan, who served as inspiration for this book and who share my fascination with kitchen and consumer product science. (Kids, sorry for such a long answer.) Thanks beyond the norm go to my wife, Gusty, who encourages and knows creativity, drive, hard work, long hours, and passion. That's what it takes. The emotional support of my family was backed up with practical sacrifices that made it all possible, to their credit. My mother applied her editorial skepticism, artfully blended with motherly encouragement, for which I'm especially grateful. (In my world, family and work go together.)

I'd like to thank my teachers, from elementary school through college, for encouraging me to investigate and to write, for which I am ever in their debt. They shaped my life. I remember each and every one of you, though I'd like especially to acknowledge Gerald Grunska for the basics and Frank Colcord, Ph.D., for encouraging my first big project.

My agent, Brian DeFiore, came on board at a key time and made this book happen. (Thanks again to my then eight-year-old, ice-cream-eating daughter, who introduced us.) And vigorous thanks are due to my dedicated, supportive, and superbly articulate editor and dynamite publisher, Laureen Rowland, whose early enthusiasm for the book and zinging editorial memos served me well over the long days and late nights it took to research and write the book. Writers need teammates like these.

One of the most important sources for the emotional fuel behind this book was the encouragement of friends, whether editorial or logistical. Included are at least these, with apologies to those not listed: Tom and Mary Kerr, Eddy and Barbara Sucherman, John and Joan Von Leesen, Jan and Stan Tymorek, William Abrams, Julie Salamon, Heidi Hansen, Heather Heath Reed, Shino Tanakawa, Jill Enfield, Richard Rabinowitz, Steven Schram, Ph.D., George LaGassa, Roy Simon, John Smallwood, David Rubel, American Book Producers Association, PS 3, and the board of PS 3 'til 6, Inc. You all supported and encouraged me in myriad ways, for which I'm especially grateful.

A note regarding those who helped me in professional capacities is found at the end of the book.

CONTENTS

Acknowledgments   *vii*

A Note to the Reader   *xiii*

1. "Where Does Polysorbate 60 Come from, Daddy?"   1

2. Wheat Flour   13

3. Bleach   21

4. Enrichment Blend: Ferrous Sulfate and
   B Vitamins—Niacin, Thiamine Mononitrate (B1),
   Riboflavin (B2), Folic Acid   29

5. Sugar   45

6. Corn Sweeteners   55

7. Corn Syrup, Dextrose, Glucose, and High Fructose
   Corn Syrup   63

8. Corn Thickeners: Cornstarch, Modified Cornstarch,
   Corn Dextrins, and Corn Flour   73

9.   Water   83

10. Soy: Partially Hydrogenated Vegetable and/or Animal
     Shortening, Soy Lecithin, and Soy Protein Isolate   87

11. Eggs   105

12. Cellulose Gum   115

13. Whey   125

14. Leavenings   133

15. Baking Soda   141

16. Phosphates: Sodium Acid Pyrophosphate and
     Monocalcium Phosphate   153

17. Salt   169

18. Mono and Diglycerides   179

19. Polysorbate 60   187

20. Natural and Artificial Flavors   199

21. Sodium Stearoyl Lactylate   215

22. Sodium and Calcium Caseinate   225

23. Calcium Sulfate   231

24. Sorbic Acid   239

25. FD&C Yellow No. 5, Red No. 40   247

26. Consider the Twinkie   257

Human Resources   265

Index   269

INGREDIENTS: ENRICHED BLEACHED WHEAT FLOUR [FLOUR, FERROUS SULFATE, "B" VITAMINS (NIACIN, THIAMINE MONO-NITRATE (B1), RIBOFLAVIN (B2), FOLIC ACID)], SUGAR, CORN SYRUP, WATER, HIGH FRUCTOSE CORN SYRUP, PARTIALLY HYDROGENATED VEGETABLE SHORTENING (CONTAINS ONE OR MORE OF: SOYBEAN, CANOLA OR PALM OIL), DEXTROSE, WHOLE EGGS. CONTAINS 2% OR LESS OF: MODIFIED CORN-STARCH, CELLULOSE GUM, WHEY, LEAVENINGS (SODIUM ACID PYROPHOSPHATE, BAKING SODA, MONOCALCIUM PHOSPHATE), SALT, CORNSTARCH, CORN FLOUR, CORN DEXTRINS, MONO AND DIGLYCERIDES, POLYSORBATE 60, SOY LECITHIN, NATUR-AL AND ARTIFICIAL FLAVORS, SOY PROTEIN ISOLATE, SODIUM STEAROYL LACTYLATE, SODUM AND CALCIUM CASEINATE, CAL-CIUM SULFATE, SORBIC ACID (TO RETAIN FRESHNESS), COLOR ADDED (YELLOW 5, RED 40). MAY CONTAIN PEANUTS OR TRACES OF PEANUTS.

Ingredient label of Hostess ® Twinkies ® "Golden Sponge Cake with Creamy Filling," purchased at the time of this writing. Ingredients, their names, and the order in which they appear vary over time and from bakery to bakery as regulations or prices or cooking techniques change.

One could be forgiven for thinking that all one might have to do to find out what goes into a Hostess® Twinkies® "Golden Sponge Cake with Creamy Filling" is to simply ask the company that makes them. But it is not that simple.

In fact, Interstate Bakeries Corporation, one of the country's largest wholesale bakeries, which owns Hostess®, Drake's® Cakes (Yodels, Devil Dogs, Yankee Doodles, and Ring Dings), Wonder® Bread, Home Pride®, Dolly Madison Bakery®, Butternut®, Merita®, and Cotton's® Holsum, among other familiar brands, was initially receptive to my requests for tours and interviews. However, after about twenty-four hours of contemplation, the company declined via phone, citing its preference to help writers who are merely reminiscing about their sweet childhood memories.

Despite this, Interstate could not have been nicer or more professional, and for that I am very grateful. Plus, I got to speak with someone who has what must be the most fabulous business title ever: Vice President of Cake. So the information on Twinkies and their ingredients comes from publicly available sources, industry professionals, and academics, but not directly from Hostess/Interstate Bakeries.

In researching this book, I traveled to see many of the ingredients' points of origin and processing myself, experiencing firsthand the alchemy of modern food science that turns recognizable commodities like corn and petroleum into anonymous white powders and viscous liquids and then turns *those* into yellow cakes with creamy filling, among many other familiar foods.

Twinkies, of course, are not the only food products made with these ingredients—they are just a perfect example. Not only do they contain many of the most common ingredients found in processed foods, they are as familiar to most consumers as a product can be. There are, in fact, some dead-on imitations: Mrs. Freshley's® Gold Creme Cakes, Little Debbie® Golden Cremes, and Lady Linda Creme Fingers, for starters (Little Debbie actually sells twice as many snack cakes, of all types, as Hostess, but because they are priced more cheaply than Twinkies, both have annual sales of around $200 million). So the functionality of each ingredient is not unique to Twinkies. The same ingredients are found in hundreds of well-known foods, such as salad dressings, ice cream, and bread—not just cakes. Surprisingly, even Ensure® nutrition shakes and toothpaste share some of these ingredients.

Many of the food scientists, food science teachers, consultants, and baking professionals I spoke with have worked on creating cakes and creamy fillings over the years for many different clients and were able to share their expertise in general terms, as the cakes all use similar ingredients, though in artfully different ways (the line between art and science is very, very thin here, as it is in most baking). Also, the ingredient and the subingredient manufacturers I spoke with were able to tell me how they make their products and how they are used with continued enthusiasm by a variety of customers, not just Interstate Bakeries. All manufacturers and processes described are examples of what is likely or typical, not exactly what is done to make Twinkies proper.

Likewise, several accomplished professionals at several different large companies in the ingredient chain offered help but only on condition of anonymity, seeking to avoid linking their companies with a specific ingredient or with Twinkies in particular. Often, my source was protecting proprietary information. For this reason, I have changed names in several places as a professional courtesy. This book does not reveal any proprietary information about Twinkies' or other companies' manufacturing nor who their suppliers are.

Any ingredient manufacturer described here may or may not supply that ingredient to Interstate Bakeries, just as they may or may not supply it to any other bakery. This is true not only because various suppliers try to keep that kind of information quiet (out of respect for their customers, among other reasons) but also because these vendor relationships change constantly. Many ingredient destinations are not traceable, as they are sold to distributors, not directly to the bakeries.

I have made every effort to be technically accurate, but because our food supply is considered vulnerable to terrorists, some location or company details have been omitted upon request. Also, the industry, recipes, and techniques are in constant flux. For these reasons, some generalities have been made. Dozens of industry professionals have reviewed the material presented here, but in the end, I am solely responsible for any errors contained herein.

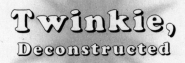

Twinkie,
Deconstructed

CHAPTER 1

"Where Does Polysorbate 60 Come from, Daddy?"

It all came to a head as I was sitting at a picnic table near the beach in Connecticut one fine August day, feeding my two little kids ice cream bars and, out of habit, casually reading the ingredient label.

"Whatcha reading, Daddy?" my six-year-old girl asked. "Uh, the ingredient label, honey. It tells us what's inside your ice cream bar." Oops. Slippery slope. Glancing back down at it, I realized it was totally incomprehensible and most terms only barely pronounceable.

"So what's in it, Dad?" asked my son, a big sixth grader, who started reading his own label aloud. "Oooooh—high fructose corn syrup! What's that? And what's pol-y-sor-bate six-tee?"

I started to sweat.

And then my sweet little girl (who at that age still thought Daddy knew everything) pitched the zinger: "Where does pol-y-sor-bate six-tee come from, Daddy?"

It was a moment of truth that every parent recognizes. When you must admit your fallibility to your worshipful children.

"Uhh . . . umm . . . I uh . . . don't have a clue, honey," was the rather disappointing—but honest—answer I mustered. Some father I was! I could speak with a fair amount of authority about Greek olives, Spanish clementines, and tuna fish. But when faced with high fructose corn syrup, I was lost.

Being a curious, food-loving guy, I actually began to think about the question more seriously. I'd always wondered what those strange-sounding ingredients were as I read labels purely out of habit, going through the motions without ever understanding or even gaining any knowledge. Then and there, I decided to put an end to the mystery and find out. I had to find the polysorbate . . . tree or wherever it came from.

※

Thinking about the origins of food is not new to me. I lived in France for six years and learned how the origin and handling of wine grapes affects how the wine tastes. I visited the actual villages that Beaujolais Villages comes from. I ate at restaurants featuring regional food—not just regional cuisine, but regional *food*. I bought locally grown fruits and vegetables, sometimes directly from the farmer at his or her farm. Now I spend most of my summers on the coast of Maine, where I can gather mussels from the nearby shore and cook them for dinner mere hours later, accompanied on occasion by fish (mackerel) we've caught and vegetables we've harvested or received from a neighbor's garden.

When you eat mussels or blueberries that you have collected yourself, or a vegetable you or a neighbor has grown, you don't have to guess where your food came from. You are consuming it as close as possible to the point of origin, reducing processing to an absolute minimum. Eat your own vegetables and fruits raw, and you've reduced "processing" to washing. Eating wild raspberries from your own yard as you pick them is about as short a link to a food source as you can get—a luscious treat and the absolute polar opposite of modern processed food. My kids don't ask me where these berries come from—they can see for themselves. At the other extreme, the point of processed food is to have no direct link to a place, or even to time. Processed food is meant to be national or even international, and the longer it remains ready for consumption the better. It's been this way since people started salting, drying, or smoking their food centuries ago.

I know from working as an assistant chef, eating at fine restaurants from time to time, and having done a few food-related books, that intriguing stories accompany many foods, stories that often deal with their origins and processing, like why some beers taste bitter while others taste malty. One glorious night a number of years ago, I was treated to a custom tasting menu by Gray Kunz, one of the best chefs in the world, at his legendary four-star restaurant, Lespinasse, in anticipation of a book project we were contemplating. One dish featured a mysterious, red, tart sauce, and in order to explain what it was made of, Chef Kunz sent out a tuxedoed waiter carrying an immense silver platter lined with sumptuous white linen upon which gently rested a little branch full of red fruit. "Mr. Kunz wanted you to see the source of this sauce—rose hips," the waiter explained.

That fateful day on the beach with my kids inspired me to do the same for Red No. 40, polysorbate 60, and mono and diglycerides. However, since I lack tuxedoed waiters on my staff, I wrote this book.

I can picture the rose hip bush whenever I see the ingredient listed somewhere, even on a jar of vitamin C (it's a great natural source). And I can tell you how and where mussels grow, and why the wines of Burgundy or the olive oils of Italy are different from those of Spain. A few years ago, I had absolutely no clue where most of the commonly used natural and artificial ingredients come from, how they are processed, how we came to think of using them in food, or what they do.

Now, I do.

✳

Instead of merely listing, in encyclopedic form, the thousands of foods and food additives that appear in the ingredient labels on products on our grocery store shelves, it seemed to make more sense to try to find a food product that embodied a number of them to serve as a prism through which to address the subject. I wanted to find a familiar food product, or even an iconic one, that many people would recognize and likely would have eaten at some point in their lives. Some kind of bread? Instant soup? Salad dressing? Yoo-hoo® Chocolate Drink? All boasted long in-gredient lists filled with compounds I didn't understand, but then I hit upon the one product that truly filled the bill. The über-iconic food product, the archetype of all processed foods, the rare food to become part of popular culture (proof: it was included in the Millennium Time Capsule by President Clinton): Twinkies®.

Twinkies' ingredient list was long enough to include a good variety of additives, including my two top targets, polysorbate 60 and high fructose corn syrup. I also liked the idea of Twinkies be-cause, along the way, I could explore some of the outlandish myths surrounding them. Twinkies are, according to urban leg-end, so full of chemicals that they will last, even exposed on a roof, for twenty-five years, and take seven years to digest. Some myths claim that they are no longer freshly baked—rather, that they were all baked decades ago—nor do they contain any actual food in them, but are the result of assorted chemical reactions. Or, as a character in a February 14, 2006, *Doonesbury* comic strip stated, baked only every February. I guessed it would be fun to see if there was any truth to these intriguing scenarios, all the while uncovering just what Twinkies are made of.

DOONESBURY

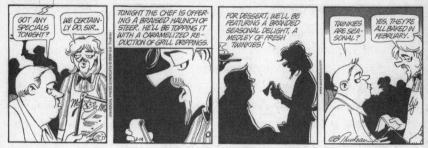

It is not clear why Twinkies may have attracted more attention than any similar snack cake. Other snack cakes use pretty much the same ingredients and strive for a similarly long or even longer shelf life—somewhere, it turns out, around twenty-five days (not years). Is it because they are blond, and denigrating blonds is another old American tradition? Is it jealousy, because they are so famous that even Archie Bunker, the main character on one of the longest-running, most popular TV shows in history (*All in the Family*) took one to lunch every day? Or does it stem from the fascination with the Twinkie's notoriety, further enshrined in the public consciousness when the innocent snack cake became unfairly ensnared in lurid headlines during the 1979 murder trial of former San Francisco City supervisor Dan White? A doctor testified that White, a normally health-conscious man, was evidently depressed because he had begun eating sugar-laden junk food. In fact, there actually was no direct link with Twinkies—it was the press that erroneously dubbed it the "Twinkie defense."

Hostess's own CupCake is actually the bestselling snack cake in history, and there are plenty of competitors just as loaded with sugar and oil that sell, in the aggregate, even more: Little Debbie®, Hostess's main competitor, puts out a long roster of sweet treats such as the aforementioned but less engagingly named Golden Cremes, and there are Ho Hos®, DingDongs®, Suzy Q's®, Devil Cremes®, Kreme Filled Krimpets®, among many other creme-filled snack cakes, but none have the allure of Twinkies. Even professional bakers casually refer to all small cakes as "Twinkies." Now *that's* an icon.

Because so many of us are disposed to believe the myths surrounding Twinkies, attempting to find the truth added even more intrigue to the investigation. The myths tie right in with the more mundane challenges posed to the bakers of such cakes: keeping the moisture balanced between the cake and the filling while it sits on a store shelf, mixing batters that can stand up to the rigors of mass production, and keeping the price low.

And so I chose the Twinkie as the vehicle for this wild trip through ingredient land—a voyage of discovery of modern food technology. The Twinkie ingredient list, printed on every package, provides the narrative structure.[1] The chapters essentially mirror the label, the ingredients in descending order of prominence, with the exception of the multiple corn and soy ingredients, which are covered in the same chapters because of their common sources and processing. Full of astonishing surprises, like how carbon monoxide plays a key role in making food additives, this journey—my journey—is the story of making convenience food, guided by science and commerce, just like the history of Twinkies themselves.

✳

While the drive to make better food goes back to the dawn of humanity, the drive to create Twinkies started during the Great

---

1. The Twinkies ingredient list, like that of other processed foods, is not etched in stone. It varies over time and even from bakery to bakery as laws (i.e., trans fats are now banned) or prices or cooking techniques change, so don't freak out if your Twinkie box doesn't match the list used here.

Depression, near Chicago. Back in 1930, James Dewar, a vice president at Continental Bakeries, bakers of Wonder® Bread and a variety of cakes, came up with a way to use the idle baking pans for Hostess's Little Shortbread Fingers, a summer strawberry treat, during their off-season. His idea, sponge cake with a creamy filling, was inexpensive enough that two cakes could sell for a nickel. Inspired by a billboard advertising "Twinkle-Toe" shoes that he passed en route to a meeting to promote his new idea, Dewar dubbed the snack cake "Twinkies." "The best darn-tootin' idea I ever had!" he is oft quoted as saying (he was widely interviewed for the cake's fiftieth anniversary in 1980). But he would soon learn that even the best darn-tootin' ideas can be fundamentally flawed.

The shelf life of the original Twinkie—two, possibly three days—posed a huge problem, a fact that dogged Dewar, according to his family. In order to maintain freshness, he had his sales reps remove unsold cakes every few days, but this was costly and inefficient. His ingredient options were also quite limited: the cake was similar to the homemade kind, as far as I can tell (no written history exists), using whole eggs for emulsifiers and lard for shortening (plus flour, water, and salt). Still, Twinkies were instantly and hugely popular, and Dewar credited this focus on freshness to his product's success. The challenge was to find a way to keep the product on the shelves longer while reducing the number of trips the salesmen (and they were all men back then) had to make to each store. With consumer products like these, shelf life is almost always a primary consideration. Even today, food scientists generally agree that aside from the overriding need to keep costs to a minimum, shelf life (cake or bread staling) is the first problem to solve. (The rather unpalatable problem of leaking moisture and fat run a close second.)

Modern food technology was Twinkies' salvation. The chemical industry worldwide exploded with innovation just after

World War II, driven in part by the war itself. Simultaneously, American demand for convenience foods (and higher profits) blossomed along with the maturing of our highway system for efficient distribution. In the 1950s, Twinkies' shelf life extended along with its ingredient list.

The result today is a cake known for its secret recipe and long shelf life. Its taste is so appealing that Hostess claims it sells 500 million a year, yet most of us don't have a clue how the Twinkie's major, basic food ingredients (wheat, sugar, soybeans, and eggs) are processed, let alone how its more unfamiliar ingredients are made—or even what they are.

✳

Understanding the ingredients in the greater context of food industry rather than simply understanding the recipe for this particular snack cake became my goal. Investigating ingredients such as sodium stearoyl lactylate or enriched, bleached flour—with ingredients coming from various states and/or foreign countries—makes you wonder why we work so hard to make any food, especially a nonnutritive snack food. After all, most of these ingredients are in the thousands of other familiar processed foods we eat, including salad dressings, sports drinks, bread, and ice cream. Examine these and you are examining much of our modern food supply.

Some ingredients, like most of those at the top of the Twinkies ingredient list, retain aspects of their agricultural origins, while others, like most of those at the bottom of the list, are either minerals or are so highly processed that they really do qualify as chemicals rather than foods. While exploring complex industrial or chemical processes, I became eager to learn how we came to know how to do this, often finding the answer rooted in history. Phosphoric acid may be an important ingredient in Coca-Cola®, but how did we come to use it in baking powder? Why did we start using chlorine for bleaching flour? What did we use in cakes before, say, polysorbate 60 or sweet dairy whey? Are any of the chemically named items extracted from vegetables or fruit? (I thought for sure something must be extracted from cranberries or tree bark, and wanted to find out.) And perhaps the most important question of all: if you can make a cake at home with just flour, sugar, butter, eggs, and water (OK, and a little flavoring, plus cream for a filling, and baking powder if you insist), how is it that thirty-nine ingredients are needed to make a Twinkie? Why do they use so many unfoodlike ingredients at all?

And then there were the intriguing, inspiring tidbits that made me want to dig even deeper, like a dictionary definition of phosphates (part of baking powder) that says, "Obtained from phosphate rock . . . Phosphorus was formerly used to treat rickets and degenerative disorders and is now used as a mineral supplement for foods; also in incendiary bombs and tracer bullets." Sure makes you wonder about what's in those cakes. Since when—and why—do we grind up rocks for food? Or, for that matter, since when do we find it necessary to reduce naturally occurring resources like corn, soybeans, and petroleum into a brown goo that is so strong in its pure form it will blow out your taste buds, yet apparently is fine to consume in cake form? How are noxious-sounding substances transformed into innocuous processed food ingredients? How is calcium sulfate (the food additive) different from calcium sulfate (the soil amendment), or from its most common form, plaster?

If you are what you eat, then it behooves you to know exactly what you are eating. Especially if you eat a lot of polysorbate 60, cellulose gum, and Red No. 40.

Finding out where, at the lowest level, these subingredients come from, tracing every finished product back down the processing chain (doing what scientists call a root tracer) is a way to give a sense of place to each ingredient. And there are some surprising stories about how each ingredient came to be made and used. Every chemical in the Twinkie comes from somewhere, and is made from things that come from somewhere else—usually from the ground. (That leads to "Aren't they all natural if they come from the earth?"—a question that dogs me still.) Organic Twinkies, not. What they are, how they are made, and how or why they are used and interact with the other ingredients are the bigger, guiding issues.

It became evident that the Twinkie is a dynamic, complex food system, where the proteins (flour, caseinates, whey, and egg) build structure and the fat and sugar (oils, emulsifiers, and sweeteners of many kinds) fight with that structure, in order to provide moisture and tenderness. Everything else on the list serves to balance out these two tendencies, some siding with moisture preservation (think "Shelf life! Shelf life!") and some helping the batter to stand up to the rigors of the commercial baking process (and to reduce overall cost). And then there's the difference between the foods at the top of the list and the chemicals at the bottom—what's that all about? Why don't I need those ingredients (calcium sulfate, sorbic acid, coloring, etc.) in my homemade cakes? Sometimes it became difficult to relate the massive industrial and technical activities involved to making the ingredients for a simple baked good. There is, in fact, quite a disconnect.

As I watched mountains being moved to get at a mineral or visited mile-long factories to see things being refined, brewed, reacted, crushed, or dried, when I began to consider the awesome number of truck, ship, and trainloads involved, when I became aware of all the cooking and slicing and dicing of molecules, I began to question how we managed to engage serious science in the pursuit of creating something that isn't even necessary to our existence. I tried to find out how we came to make food additives on a global scale, and I had to wonder why we make such an enormous industrial effort to create artificial replacements for relatively unprocessed things like sugar. I wondered where this industry fit in with the major industries of the world.

And, from the start, I wanted to know: when can I go see where they come from?

CHAPTER 2

Wheat Flour

Flour, along with fat and sugar, is what defines a cake. Every other ingredient—including those infamous chemicals—is in the recipe to help make the flour into something light, tasty, and a delight to eat. But flour is the base. Believers of urban legend, take note: Twinkies are not just made of chemicals. They are made mostly from flour, one of the most important and ancient foods we eat. That's why flour is first on the ingredient list, and the first ingredient I explore.

For many of the Twinkies bakeries around the country, wheat for their cake flour comes from traditional, family farms like those in what the farmers call the Delmarva area (short for Delaware Maryland Virginia). A typical farm is the one thousand acres in Queen Anne, Maryland, that Jimmy Boyle's family has farmed for generations. Thanks to modern combines (harvester/planter machines) and other high-tech equipment, he can farm his land with only a couple of helpers, delivering wheat by truck to a nearby grain elevator, which acts as a dealer and sells the wheat to the big eastern flour mills. The favorable climate allows Boyle to grow three crops on the same land every two years by rotating with corn and soybeans. Maximum return for maximum effort. Boyle keeps his land busy.

The relatively small size of the farms in this area is what creates the alluring patchwork pattern of fields in much of the mid-Atlantic and eastern part of the Midwest, and its beauty is what cheers me as I drive to one of the biggest flour mills in the country to see wheat milled into cake flour for Twinkies.

The genial wheat and baking expert I meet there is eager to explain everything about the process to me, but his employers are slow to respond to his enthusiasm. He decides to show me around anyhow (while keeping certain rooms and information off-limits), as long as he and his conglomerate-like company remain nameless. For the purposes of this narrative, I'll call him Bob Alexander.

Every spring, Alexander tours hundreds of traditional, small family farms like Boyle's in eastern Pennsylvania, western New Jersey, and the Delaware-Maryland peninsula. He's a total professional, and loves the science and art of baking (and loves talking about it). A man on a mission, he travels the fields to test and find the proper wheat to turn into Twinkies. Some of the farms are Amish, which provides a nice irony: the arch nonconsumers supplying the arch consumers.

On a typical visit, Alexander measures the protein, starch, and moisture content of each farm's soft red winter wheat, the wheat used for cake flour. Nature is inconsistent, but the Twinkie recipe must be respected, so Alexander examines and travels and talks and buys and hopes to get to the best crops before his several competitors do. Most of what he reveals paints a surprisingly complex image of what most of us take for granted as plain old flour, a common kitchen staple. But like everything else in Twinkies, just because it is common doesn't make it simple.

SOFT RED

Turns out, wheat is not just wheat. There are six kinds, and each varies in moisture and in gluten, the primary protein complex in wheat and the main thing that influences how it functions in a particular recipe. Gluten—and the proportion of it found in each kind of wheat—is what makes certain types of wheat better and more appropriate for various uses. Hard red spring and hard red winter wheats (high-gluten/high-protein wheats from the vast wheat fields of the northern Great Plains) are used for bread and pizza flour; hard white (from California and Kansas) makes good bread flour. Soft white (from northern New York and the Northwest) is best for noodle and cracker flour. Durum (extra hard, from the north central states) is used for pasta flour. And soft red winter wheat, from the mid-Atlantic (i.e., Jimmy Boyle's farm), South, and Ohio and Mississippi River valleys, makes the best cake flour.

Twinkies (according to Hostess) consume 7 million pounds of this flour yearly. That's 3.5 million of the two-pound bags of flour you buy at the grocery store.

Cake flour, by definition, is milled from soft, low-protein, high-starch wheat that absorbs very little water. Because it has the lowest protein of all wheats (7 to 9 percent in cake flour versus 12 to 14 percent for bread flour) and thus a low gluten content, it works best with almost equal amounts of sugar and the heavy emulsifiers, which blend the oil and water. The flour, which is ground much finer than regular wheat, is perfect for Twinkies and their high-volume, fine-textured, delicate crumb. But cake flour's low protein can also be too much of a good thing—some cake recipes actually have to add a bit of powdered wheat gluten, not only to strengthen the weak flour, but as a stabilizer and thickener as well as to add some smoothness to the cake's inside and surface.

Flour professionals sneer at the consumer's trusty standby,

"All-Purpose" flour blend, which varies in its blend from brand to brand and region to region. "It's good for nothing if it says 'good for everything,'" Alexander snorts, while standing in the midst of the giant mill where he works. Dough made from high-gluten (high-protein) flour, like pizza dough, is cake flour's polar opposite: its texture, made tough from all that protein, means it can stretch and hold big bubbles of gas without much more than water and yeast.

GRINDING GRASS

Wheat, which is a grass, looks like regular lawn grass for most of its life. When Boyle harvests it with his giant combine, the bushy top, which holds the seeds (called wheat kernels or wheat berries) is removed and collected. Twinkies literally start here, in the field.

The stems are dried for straw (hay is made from another kind of grass) and the grain is conveyed from the top of the combine into a grain truck, which looks like a normal semi but for the big udders (hanging from its bottom, where the grain is discharged), and its convertible, canvas top. These trucks deliver and sell grain to a local co-op, or to a group of storage silos owned by a dealer who in turn sells it to a big food processing company like Con-Agra, Archer Daniels Midland (ADM), or Cargill. Around flour mills located in urban areas, you can spot spilled wheat berries on city streets. Rural grist for urban mills.

Wheat stores well. At the big flour mill I visit, there is a wall of office-building-size storage silos out behind the main plant, each of which holds half a million bushels of grain, 150 railroad cars' worth. The scale stems from the need for tons of backup grain to keep the huge mill functioning in case of any interruption in supply. Plus, of course, wheat is a seasonal crop. Still, that is one mighty big wall.

Wheat milling began, old pros like to say, when some prehistoric soul wandering through a grass field took a bite of a raw wheat berry. If it was soft red winter wheat, it was soft enough to chew, and the first evolutionary step toward civilization and Twinkie-making was taken. (If it was hard winter wheat, it felt like chomping down on a pebble, and no progress was made, except possibly toward the invention of dentistry.) Early millers, as far back as 6700 (some say 7500) BC, simply pounded the berries with smooth stones, something primitive people still do today in preparation for their daily meals. Ever since fully mechanized flour mills became popular in the early 1800s, and especially since the invention of the superefficient roller mill in 1879, mass consumers have been convinced that whiter, finer flour was the way to go, setting the stage for Twinkies.

Today, modern millers erect multimillion-dollar mills to mill the wheat berries—a process of seventy to eighty mechanical steps overall, making the finest flour a baker could ask for, at least for making Twinkies. The mill itself (which I have agreed not to identify, but which is similar to the others I have visited) is an agglomeration of different kinds of buildings, including a small clump of ten-story-tall, cylindrical silos made of cement. Like most mills, it is well served by a country road as well as by a rail line. There's lots of pavement out front—parking for dozens of open-topped grain trucks and tank-like, cylindrical flour trucks suggests urban congestion in an otherwise fairly rural area. Conveyors, some caged in steel latticework, others in enclosed boxy shafts, tie the bigger buildings and silos together. And the squat, steel grain storage silos out back provide a visual balance to the slender cement silos out front. A white, cement office building that houses a dozen workers appears only as an afterthought.

The place is easier to get into if you're driving a sixteen-wheeler than if you happen to be in an old Ford Taurus station wagon. I have to steer carefully, skirting the trucks and their giant loading bays, way to the side and around out back, to find my way to the office. The grain—the talent, if you will—is escorted briskly back.

The mill is full of noisy rooms spread among several tall buildings. The wheat berries travel through a wide variety of machines, including separators (sticks and stones may break your mill); aspirators (to suck up dust and dirt); a scourer (to get some roughage—outer husks—and more dirt off); a washer-stoner (to remove more dirt and stones); a few seed separators; then water-filled tempering bins to soften the inner part (the endosperm, the source of flour) and toughen the outer part (the bran) for easier separation; and finally, as many as twelve steps just for grinding and sifting. This is not a simple process, though no chemicals are involved.

The room full of roller milling machines looks somewhat like a Laundromat gone wild. The machines—disarmingly small, waist-high, and three to six feet wide—are lined neatly in long rows; metal and plastic pneumatic tubes veer off the tops every which way, constantly circulating and recirculating the flour until it is ground just right. Resistance is futile. Big mills like this one often have fifty or sixty milling machines; smaller ones only twenty.

These are precision instruments, and the best are manufactured in Switzerland. Each machine has a little, laptop-like control panel and a long, clear plastic lid that the technicians can lift for sampling. The rollers—a pair to each milling machine—are narrow, grooved, and cooled stainless steel rods that spin in a noisy whir. One moves a bit faster than the other, producing a shearing action where the berry or part of a berry is caught between them, breaking the center (endosperm) from the exterior (bran), and giving this first device the name "breaker mill."

The few guys wandering out from the control room wear ear

protectors. A thin coat of white dust graces the floor, softening the angles of the machines throughout the mill. The air/flour mixture flows like water, sending the acceptable grains on and the larger ones back for another grind through what amounts to thousands of hissing tubes that crisscross the plant. In just one small, three-foot square, I count eight tubes passing through the floor. The triage is constant, the flow is continuous, and the dust vacuums hum loudly.

No one smokes in a flour mill—flour dust, like any organic (carbon-based) dust, is explosive. Add a tiny spark from a motor, static electricity, or worse, a welding torch, and *kaBOOM*! (As a result, all repairs are done when the plant is "down.")

The same danger is especially high where other crops with carbohydrates in them are milled or processed: cocoa, cotton, sugar, and, of course, wood. Other explosive foods are custard powder, instant coffee, dried milk, potato powder, and soup powder. Even metal dusts can explode. It is hard to imagine that these simple and common products, lurking on our shelves as we sleep, are capable of blowing their processing plants to smithereens.

Every point where flour dust could escape is designed to minimize the risk of explosion. Vacuums are the first line of defense, and some areas feature negative air pressure, so dust clouds can't form. The doors close and seal tightly to maintain high air pressure, and casual visitors are unwelcome (I'm personally guided and wearing a bright red, color-coded hard hat indicating my security clearance).

Other than Alexander and me, there seem to be only a few technicians in the plant. This is one of the most automated of professions—the first fully automated manufacturing process in history, industry organizations are fond of boasting—and it seems appropriate, this modern melding of industry and agriculture. Flour is one of the very basic foodstuffs. It is the primary ingredient in the staff of life as well as the stuff of Twinkies. But there is a lot more to cake flour than just ground-up grass, probably a lot more than you ever imagined. Before it can be shipped out, it requires the addition of bleach (yes, bleach) and vitamins, both of which are completely industrial products, in stark contrast to their natural, grassy partner.

CHAPTER 3

Bleach

When my kids ask me if the same bleach we use on our laundry is used to bleach flour, I have to say, "Well, yes, sort of." "Eeewwww" is the studied (and, let's face it, expected) response. Household bleach and flour bleach share the same essential ingredient—chlorine. That must mean that Twinkie flour—that nice, clean, familiar cake flour—is then bleached with poisonous chlorine gas. But don't worry, it's OK to eat (we think). It's just hard to see where it's made. To make chlorine for bleaching cake flour or disinfecting water or making plastic pipes, you need just two raw ingredients: tons of salt and a whole lot of electricity. And both salt and hydroelectric power are found in abundance around Niagara Falls, New York.

The chloralkali, or chlor/alkali, industry—that's the term for chlorine makers—is one of the largest industries in the world, and chlorine is the tenth most common chemical made in the United States, so a lot of companies should be making chlorine up there, and were, until a few years ago. One would think it would be easy to find a few giant chlorine companies, but many of the people in the flour industry who use it are unable to say where it is made or by whom. It turns out that most have gone out of business (strange, given that chlorine is such a commonly used chemical) or have merged into various conglomerates (alas, not as strange). Many were victims, to be sure, of bad management, but safety and other government regulations have no doubt taken their toll on the smaller players.

I did find two very helpful companies, though. Nearly a hundred years ago, predecessors of what is now OxyChem®, Occidental Petroleum Corporation's chemical subsidiary, the largest merchant marketer of chlorine in the United States, located what is now one of its biggest plants in the previously mentioned area of Niagara Falls, New York. PPG Industries, formerly Pittsburgh Plate Glass, has one across the nearby border, in Beauharnois, near Montreal, and several on the Gulf Coast, notably Lake Charles, Louisiana, and Beaumont, Texas. These plants either sit directly atop salt deposits (as in the Gulf Coast, where most of our chlorine is now produced) or next to inexpensive hydropower (Quebec). Chlorine industry spokespeople claim that they use 1 percent of the electricity generated in the United States, to make approximately 26 *billion* pounds of chlorine each year. They also say that they use 44 billion pounds of table salt to do this, enough to cover, in one of the more imaginative metaphors ever conceived, almost three hundred large orders of french fries for each American, every day.

The term "chloralkali" is deeply rooted in language, not science. The word "chlorine" itself comes from Greek for "greenish yellow," a name chosen by British chemist Sir Humphry Davy in 1810, when he determined that chlorine was an element. (It had first been isolated thirty-six years earlier, in 1774, by Swedish chemist Carl Wilhelm Scheele.) The root of the word "alkali" is *al-qili*, which is Arabic for "plant ashes," the source of what has been known since antiquity as the common household alkali chemical lye—sodium or potassium hydroxide. The ancient recipe is simply thoroughly washed plant ashes (though "lye" is from Latin for "wash," it is not a stretch to suggest that it might come from the last syllable of that Arabic word as well).

Separating Salt

Finding the chlorine companies might have been a bit difficult, but getting inside them proved impossible. Normally, no one can casually visit a chlorine plant, not even a food or science writer, nor (presumably) any potential terrorists. The intricacies of chlorine manufacturing are complicated by the fact that this is a secretive industry, for national security as well as for competitive reasons, in addition to the fact that chlorine is seriously toxic.

Despite having befriended some helpful employees who strived to get me in (my high-management level OxyChem contact—let's call him Pedro Gonzales—tried hard; others were candidly pessimistic), no dice. Typically the companies offer only general scientific information. You won't find many glorious pictures of their plants on their Web sites or in their annual reports, but part of the reason for that is also because the equipment is quite prosaic. Most sites feature a combination of boxy steel buildings surrounded by refinery-like towers, a web of pipes, and busy railroad sidings. Terry Smith, Director of Technology for PPG Industries, chuckles as he points out the chlorine building at one big chemical plant (full of intimidating towers and pipes that I hoped were for making the gas) as the one building that looks exactly like every nondescript warehouse in the world—a plain old box. Even their industry association is vague on details. The plants can be especially dangerous—that's the national security deal—because chlorine gas is absolutely deadly, which is why it and other toxic gases were used in World War I to fill the trenches and kill masses of soldiers. The results were so awful that the use of any gas as a weapon, including chlorine, was banned by the Geneva Conventions and the more recent Chemical Weapons Convention. Lucky for us and for Twinkies, chlorine is only part of a minor chemical reaction in cake flour, not an ingredient you ingest. But still.

From what I'm told by Smith and other industry experts, you can't smell any chlorine in the plant, which is not only reassuring but almost astounding: it's detectable by the human nose at only one part per million (1 ppm). Gonzales tells me you can smell more bleach in your laundry room than in a chlorine plant, which, of course, begs the question, "Why?" Smith explains, with an engineer's stoicism, "You don't want to release any chlorine. We just don't allow it. You design for that." What that means, among other things, is that if the plant should experience a power interruption, the cells shut down and the scrubbers absorb chlorine into the caustic soda also made there, which instantly creates something akin to household bleach. Gonzales is proud to point out that this also means that working in some chlorine plants is safer, by OSHA standards, than working in a commercial bank. Pick your poison.

My son's chemistry class began exploring the periodic table as I began writing this chapter, and his teacher referenced chlorine as an example of an element easily found at home—which is true, just not in pure form. Chlorine may be one of the twelve most common elements in the earth, but it is always found naturally combined with something else, like sodium, with which it forms salt (sodium chloride, or $NaCl$). These days chlorine is made by releasing it from salt in an electrochemical reaction called electrolysis, the one first envisioned by the English chemist Michael Faraday in his early experiments with electricity in the mid-1800s and often studied or demonstrated in chemistry classrooms. The modern, current form of electrolysis—which coincidently makes sodium hydroxide—became the norm for chlorine production only when electricity became available to industry. The first plant to use it, in 1893, was in Rumford, Maine.

At a typical plant—and, for homeland security reasons, I have been asked to not specifically identify one—the brine (concentrated salt water) is pumped into fiberglass and/or titanium electrochemical cells in a room the size of a typical high school gymnasium. Each cell, and there may be up to a hundred in a room, appears to be about the size of a couple of good-size deep freezers, about eight feet long by four feet wide and high. The room holds a daunting maze of hundreds of brine pipes and electrical conduits laid out flat, in a kind of rectangular city. Two thick copper bars carry massive amounts of current to electrodes in each cell's side, and various pipes and tubes channel a continuous supply of salt water. The cells seem happy enough with their plight: they hum as they work.

It may be simple chemistry, but it's still a little dangerous. It starts with a tank of salt water and a strong electrical current, which causes the chlorine to separate from the sodium in the salt and gather at one side, while the hydrogen separates from the oxygen in the water and scurries to the other side, a bit like two boxers after the bell rings. What's left behind is sodium hydroxide, also known as caustic soda, which plays an important role in making at least seven Twinkie ingredients common among all processed foods, including sodium caseinate, sodium stearoyl lactylate, artificial colors, corn flour, soybean oil, vegetable shortening, and soy protein isolate. Whether or not you can pronounce 'em, it's all in the family.

The two gases, chlorine and hydrogen,[2] are carefully kept apart for good reason. If they were to be exposed to sunlight together in just the right conditions, they could explode.

---

2. Some hydrogen is burnt with chlorine to make hydrochloric acid (HCl), an important part of a bunch of other food ingredient recipes.

PIPES AND CAKE

The elemental chlorine, Cl_2, is piped out as a greenish yellow gas, which is further purified, compressed, and liquefied at extreme subzero temperatures. Most plants use the bulk of it right there to make other things, like vinyl siding or plastic pipe, aka PVC (polyvinylchloride), a far cry from bread and cake, or so you thought. The rest is often just piped directly into pressurized, extrasecure train cars or neighboring chemical plants. Astonishingly important, chlorine is essential to about half of all chemicals made by the chemical industry, and about 85 percent of all pharmaceuticals. It is used to purify about 98 percent of our drinking water, too (and to keep our swimming pools clean). On top of all this, chlorine plays a common, useful, and helpful role in our daily diet.

When it comes to flour, fresher is not better. In fact, for centuries, freshly milled flour was stored for a few months in order to allow for natural oxidation before it was sold. Oxidation whitened the flour, which starts out a creamy yellow thanks to the natural yellow-orange carotenoid pigments found in wheat—the source of the image "amber waves of grain." By the late 1800s, consumers had started paying higher prices for whiter flour. Manufacturers responded, naturally, by looking for more efficient, less costly ways to meet that demand (time is money).

In 1879, two important developments occurred to bring us closer to the perfection of cake flour and the birth of Twinkies. The UK Patent Office (one of the oldest in the world) granted a patent for using chlorine as a bleaching agent, and modern roller mills were introduced. Soon after, in the early 1900s, when chlorine gas first became widely available in the United States, millers found that they could duplicate the three-month, natural maturation process in only a matter of seconds by pumping minute amounts of chlorine gas (less than 25 ppm) into the flour, simultaneously achieving three results: bleaching; oxidation (taming the protein or starch to the point where it is practically nonfunctional, so as to yield bread and cakes with a soft, delicate crumb); and balancing (reducing the pH by generating just a bit of hydrochloric acid to further tame the protein). Once this became evident, in 1912, chlorination started in earnest.

It is not clear exactly how this all works; what is clear is that this treatment makes bleached flour the only kind that works in sugar-heavy and "high-ratio" (more sugar than flour) cakes like Twinkies or birthday and wedding cakes. Not only do you not need chlorinated flour to make bread, you don't want it—chlorination knocks out gluten's strength. Cakes made with unbleached flour and approximately equal amounts of sugar, like pound cakes, tend to be heavier, coarser, or denser than tender sponge cakes. In other words, no chlorine, no Twinkie.

PIG IN A POKE

Because it is so dangerous, chlorine for bleaching flour is usually shipped in accident- and bullet-proof, seven-foot-long pressurized tanks called pigs. They are so heavily constructed—some of the steel is 1.5 inches thick—that an empty one-ton (2,000-pound) capacity tank actually weighs 1,500 pounds.

When the chlorine-filled pigs are finally delivered to Alexander's flour mill, they are penned in a tiny, specially constructed, high-security, negative air pressure, hazardous material bungalow. A timid glance inside reveals that they look especially small and unassuming for something so potentially dangerous. And the chlorine just barely trickles out of the pigs into the mill, where it is fed into an agitator, the last step in the milling process. This agitator is not a political troublemaker, but rather a seven-foot-long, submarine-like mixing container. The flour is pushed through it by five-inch-long, maple paddles that fluff up the flour to keep it airborne so that it can mix easily and continually with the chlorine gas being sprayed in. In this otherwise stainless steel world, wooden paddles are one of the few things that stand up to the highly corrosive chlorine. The reaction is instant, and the flour emerges properly bleached and acid-balanced after only a few seconds. The now white flour shoots out a large tube over our heads and out across the road to the blending building to become enriched with vitamins, the final treatment before it can be used in cakes.

The short story is that the mill has to put back into the flour what it took out of it, plus a little extra for good measure (and good health). The long story is that it has to go all around the world to get what it needs.

CHAPTER 4

Enrichment Blend: Ferrous Sulfate and B Vitamins— Niacin, Thiamine Mononitrate (B1), Riboflavin (B2), Folic Acid

In 1915, ten thousand people in the United States died of pellagra. If you haven't heard of pellagra or anyone dying of it lately, that is thanks largely to enriched flour. If everyone ate a well-balanced diet, or used only whole wheat flour, and/or took vitamin supplements whenever they were needed, enrichment—the process of adding back vitamins and minerals to foods from which they were removed—would become unnecessary and obsolete. (Fortification—adding vitamins and minerals to foods that don't normally have them—is a different animal.)

In 1938, the U.S. government realized it could fight pellagra, beriberi, iron deficiency anemia, and other diseases by fortifying commonly consumed foods with nutrients in the form of vitamins and a mineral (iron). Because flour was not only the most commonly eaten food in America at that time, but also one that was easily modified, and because industrial manufacturing of some vitamins had recently become a commercial reality, on January 1, 1942, the FDA simply directed the flour mills to add certain vitamins and minerals to white flour (an inexpensive national health plan without angst). The list hasn't changed since then except in 1998, when folic acid was mandated for inclusion in the mix as a means of preventing spina bifida and other defects of the brain and spinal cords of developing fetuses.

While people learned, over the ages, to treat certain diseases with specific foods—night-blindness with liver, scurvy with citrus or pine needle extracts—it wasn't until 1912 that the concept of vitamins was conceived. Polish biochemist Casimir Funk coined the name "vital amines" (*amine* is the chemical term for something made from ammonia and containing nitrogen) while he was trying to isolate the "anti-beriberi factor" from brown rice (this was based on the observation that people who ate brown rice seemed immune to the disease, while those who ate white rice weren't). Somehow the words got combined, the *e* got dropped (when it was discovered that not all of them were amines), and an industry was born. All thirteen vitamins were discovered by 1948 and synthesized by 1972.

As simple and inexpensive as enrichment seems, there is a catch: it is hard to make vitamins and minerals. Research into how best to manufacture them simply and cleanly takes years and millions of dollars. Patents and secret processes abound. The factories are complex and require specialized raw ingredients. The actual chemical synthesis of vitamins might be quick, but it is dirty, and it is a challenge to handle the nasty solvents and waste products involved. Cutting-edge biotechnology and genetic engineering are central (fermentation, the biotech route, is overtaking chemical synthesis as the way to go). And the companies aren't talking—months of dead-end research proves that. It is virtually impossible to find anyone who will explain the manufacturing process, which changes daily and therefore leads to a lot of false information. Especially galling is that the multinational companies that claim to make the vitamins are changing so fast that even they don't know, or won't say with any authority, who makes what.[3]

Some of the flux is typical, but, nevertheless, it's not good business. In 1999, the six major vitamin companies that controlled 80 percent of the world market were caught in a price-fixing scandal, the billion-dollar settlement of which led to the disappearance of some, the mergers of others (Dutch giant DSM, the world's largest vitamin manufacturer, paid more than a billion dollars to acquire Hoffman–La Roche's vitamin business in 2003), and a huge drop in prices (in the neighborhood of 75 to 80 percent). Between the penalties and the price drop, the business became a burden for most of the big Western companies. BASF, the other giant, has started several "joint ventures" in Japan and China since 2001 that even it seems to find difficult to identify. Because of the price-fixing lawsuit, and because the Western world has intensified its pollution laws (vitamin manufacturing can take a heavy environmental toll), the industry is moving quickly to countries such as India and especially China. Most of the minor players seem to have joint ventures or distribution deals of various sorts that allow them to call themselves manufacturers when all they really do is resell Chinese chemicals—a far cry from the farmer's market.

It is likely that most of us, as I did before starting this book, think that vitamins are squeezed from fruits or somehow extracted from vegetables. That's where our mothers told us to get them, after all, and eating naturally vitamin-rich foods is still the best way. But, in fact, it is actually harder to extract B vitamins from natural sources than it is to create them synthetically. Even though they are chemically identical, lab-made vitamins are better because they are consistent in strength and quality, while the

---

3. Most of the professionals asked to name the vitamin manufacturers actually cite a company that has been defunct for several years, hardly a reassuring element in the food-processing picture.

amount of a vitamin in each of several pieces of fruit, for example, varies widely with the crop and storage specifics, how much you eat, and how well your meals are balanced.

So eating a little enriched white flour isn't necessarily a bad idea—and in the United States, it's your only option.

The B vitamins in enriched flour come from elemental ores, petroleum, bacteria, or fungi made in ways you would never allow in your house. Some are a total chemical synthesis, and some are fermented. There are four vitamins and one mineral in the enriched flour that's used in Twinkies, and they don't grow in the local wheat fields. Most of them come from lands far, far away: Switzerland and China. Iron, the lone mineral, is the only one that can still come from the States, and has a popular foreign alternative.

FERROUS SULFATE: IRON SALT AND PICKLE LIQUOR

The touch of iron in a Twinkie usually begins not only in iron ore mines in Minnesota, which is no surprise, but also in oil wells, which is.

Sulfate, as the name suggests, is derived from sulfur, which is no longer mined but instead refined out of high-sulfur ("sour") crude oil, a step developed primarily to lessen air pollution when the oil is burned. Almost all of the refineries around the country, such as those near the Gulf Coast, buy crude oil from sources around the world, remove sulfur as a gas, liquefy it into elemental sulfur, and ship it at just below 300°F if by truck, or in steam-jacketed rail cars if by train (it has to be heated up and remelted at the destination) to sulfuric acid manufacturers. Most acid plants are located near the refineries. Giant chemical conglomerates DuPont and Rhodia are the leading manufacturers, with their biggest plants in Houston, Texas, and Baton Rouge,

Louisiana. These acid companies in turn burn the sulfur to get sulfur dioxide (some sulfur dioxide is used to process corn into syrup and starch) and then pass that gas over racks of expensive vanadium catalysts in building-size towers and mix it with water to get sulfuric acid. Sulfuric acid is part of the processing of a number of unrelated Twinkie subingredients (phosphoric acid, lactic acid) and one ingredient (artificial vanilla), but contributes sulfur directly only to one: ferrous sulfate.

At 165 million tons per year, sulfuric acid is the most produced chemical in the world. The United States is the world leader, making about a quarter of that sum. It is so useful that it plays a role in just about everything that's manufactured, from fertilizers to gasoline, including Twinkies. But the workers at the wells, refineries, acid plants, and steel mills haven't an inkling that what they're producing actually ends up in food.

＊

In a Midwestern steel mill, iron ore is baked and reacted into steel and then squeezed into continuous thin sheets up to 1,400 feet long in hot rolling mill lines that look like oversize printing presses. The buildings can stretch to a mile long. A rusty, crusty, oxide scale forms immediately on the surface of the fresh steel and must be removed quickly by what is known as the pickling process, which doesn't have much to do with vinegar and cucumbers. Still, it is part of a small food chain that links petroleum to a vitamin supplement to nutritious flour. Steel pickling involves running that continuous sheet through sulfuric acid in tubs up to eighty feet long and seven feet wide. The acid is known as the pickle liquor, one liquor that is not recommended for consumption but that plays a key role in making ferrous sulfate for Twinkies.

At the end of the day, after thousands of feet of steel roll have been run through the tub (impressively named "deep tank technology") and rolled into the six-foot-wide, seven-foot-diameter rolls you see carried on flatbed trucks, the sulfuric acid has become saturated with iron and is pumped out for separation. Iron sulfate crystals, an iron salt of sulfuric acid, drop to the bottom so that the acid can be poured off and recycled for further pickling. The crystals are then partially dried into dark, sandy clumps, and shipped by the truckload to the ferrous sulfate processors in one-ton supersacks.

The biggest ferrous sulfate processor in the United States, by far, and one that specializes in the purest food-grade additive, is Crown Technology in Indianapolis, Indiana, according to their VP of Operations, J. Scott Peterson. Crown dries and purifies the crystals from Midwestern steel mills and grinds them into a metallic gray powder, shipping many thousands of pounds a day in fifty-pound boxes. The finest, most consistent particles are sent to flour enrichment companies like those that supply Hostess.

Much of their ferrous sulfate is used in nonnutritious ways, products and processes that include fabric dye, ink, water purification, wood preservation, and weed killers. But fortification is also a lucrative business, and the next big thing seems to be adding iron to tortillas in order to fight rampant anemia in Mexico.

Twinkie bakeries sometimes switch between reduced iron and ferrous sulfate (FS), probably based more on pricing and availability than on nutrition or chemistry. Reduced iron is made from food-quality iron that has been reacted with carbon monoxide and/or hydrogen to get ferric oxide (technically the same as rust) that is then ground into an ultrafine, dustlike powder. Reduced iron is less expensive but not as strong as ferrous sulfate; the more finely it is ground, the more digestible, but also the more expensive it becomes. This said, it comes mostly from India and China, where labor costs are dramatically lower than in the United States, so cost is an issue vaguely in its favor.

Reduced iron is also less likely than FS to cause rancidity in fat.

There are some negatives, though: its little specks might darken the Twinkies, and when flour companies pass their product through strong magnets, looking for errant nuts, bolts, or wedding rings, it's possible that the reduced iron dust might pop out, which would be embarrassingly counterproductive, to say the least.

Niacin (B3): Alpine Oil

Niacin is made a world away from Midwestern steel mills. In Switzerland, on the Lonza River just a bit north of the Matterhorn, not far from Zermatt, in the little Alpine valley town of Visp (population about 6,600), window boxes overflow with bright flowers. Perfectly squared-off farms frame the village border. Snow-covered Alps hover nearby. And Lonza Ltd. makes most of the world's niacin in an ultraclean liquefied petroleum gas (LPG)/naphtha cracker and petrochemical plant, a mini-city of orderly tubes, towers, and huge tanks surrounded by squiggly white and green pipes and covered with catwalks and ladders.

Lonza's Director of Nutrition, Elias Alonso, the only vitamin manufacturer to offer me a tour, explains the complex processing of simple ingredients. Water and air are two of the three basic ingredients of niacin (water and air are the definition of basic). The third is petroleum, in the form of naphtha or liquid petroleum gas, which is culled from the Middle East or the North Sea and then processed by French and Italian refineries. All together, these three seem an unlikely mix of raw ingredients for a vitamin. First, the petroleum is cracked (processed under extreme heat and pressure) into methane (which leads to acetylene, as in welding torches), ethylene (which goes on to make the common plastic polyethylene as well as a zillion other things), and hydrogen. Air is liquefied and distilled to separate the nitrogen from the oxygen. The nitrogen is mixed with hydrogen (from natural gas) under high heat and pressure to make ammonia, which is then mixed with oxygen blown through a platinum gauze in order to make nitric acid (that's the source of the nitrogen, the original "amine" that led to the discovery of all vitamins). The ethylene and acetylene are then mixed under pressure with some water and a rare platinum catalyst to make acetaldehyde, a flammable liquid, which is further processed and mixed with ammonia. It doesn't seem very healthy or remotely digestible at this point, but eventually, in a neat bit of forward planning (which is curiously called "backward integration"), some of the previously manufactured nitric acid is mixed with ammonia/acetaldehyde blend resulting in niacin, a white solid that is milled into a flourlike powder and packed into twenty-kilogram bags.

Vitamin B3 is one of the few vitamins that the body can make, which it does with more finesse than the Swiss by converting the amino acid tryptophan, commonly found in fish, lean meat, whole grains, and, of course, turkey. However, you'd need to consume much more than you normally eat to fight pellagra, that old-fashioned disease that boasts a whole range of symptoms including severe dermatitis, diarrhea, dementia, and death (perhaps niacin should be called the anti-D vitamin).

Pellagra was common in Europe and Central America for two hundred years, and in the rural South of the United States after the Civil War, when cornmeal, which does not contain niacin, became a food staple, along with salt pork and molasses. A more varied diet would have prevented the problem, but farmers at this time were concentrating on cash crops like cotton and tobacco, not food. In the United States, especially in the poor South, pellagra claimed more lives than any other nutritional deficiency—more than 100,000 just since 1900. Niacin fortification simply eliminated pellagra as a death threat. Also, it's important to note that niacin alone is not only essential for growth and energy, the other B vitamins actually cannot function properly without it.

Thiamine Mononitrate (B1): The First One

Although natural thiamine is found in small quantities in many foods, it is the husk of brown rice that led to its discovery; in fact, it was the first vitamin to be discovered at all. Christiaan Eijkman, a Dutch scientist who worked in Indonesia, realized in the late 1800s that only those people eating polished (white rice) from which the brown husk—the rice bran—had been removed suffered from the awful, nerve-damaging disease beriberi. ("Beriberi," a Sinhalese word meaning "I cannot, I cannot," became the name of the disease because a victim is too sick to do anything due to extreme stiffness of the lower limbs, pain, and even paralysis.) By isolating the factor that was essential to health in this one case, Eijkman concluded that certain chemicals in food were essential to health in general, laying the groundwork for the discovery of vitamins (and a Nobel Prize in Medicine in 1929) a few years later.

In 2005, the world's largest fine chemical company, the German firm BASF, started a cooperative Chinese venture with the Tianjin Zhongjin Pharmaceutical Co., a couple of hours north of Beijing, creating what is now the world's largest B1 plant. Each year, BASF expects to produce three thousand tons of a material that is used by the fraction of an ounce in pills and, of course, bread, pasta, and Twinkies.

The manufacturing process of thiamine varies from company to company and is an especially closely guarded secret. But thiamine mononitrate, the most common form of thiamine, is usually synthesized from basic petrochemicals derived from that old trusted food source, coal tar. Thiamine chemicals are finished with about fifteen steps that may include, depending on the company, such appetizing processes as oxidation with corrosive strength hydrogen peroxide and active carbon; reactions with ammonium nitrate, ammonium carbonate, and nitric acid (to form a salt); and washing with alcohol. It is edible at this point, but before it can be mixed into flour, the manufacturer dries it into crystals and sieves it into a fine powder. Some is further reacted with methanol, hydrochloric acid, and ethanol to make thiamine hydrochloride, another popular version of thiamine found in packaged foods.

Riboflavin (B2): Brewed to Perfection

Great chefs each have their own signature way of roasting chicken or making french fries, and all the giant vitamin companies have their own, usually patented, ways of making riboflavin, also known as vitamin B2. A few make it from chemical synthesis, but most ferment it from a microorganism: yeast, a fungus, or bacteria. Candida yeasts are common; *Ashbya gossypii* fungus is used to make about 30 percent of the world's supply of B2; and some of the biggest producers favor a bacteria called *Bacillus subtilis*. Some make it from spent beer grain, recycled by the beer companies. In nature, B2 comes from leafy green veggies, liver, fish, milk, and poultry. In manufacturing, it might be fair to say that the vitamin is extracted from natural sources (these microorganisms are all natural to soil), but it is not quite that simple.

Generally the Chinese vitamin companies ferment riboflavin by putting what they call the "master organism" in a stew of various fats or carbohydrates along with some vitamins and minerals and a combination of temperatures and air in ways that vary from place to place as much as cooking technique might vary from chef to chef. With fats, it might be a stinky mix of nutrient-rich waste fats, or cod liver oil or canola or soybean oil. As when making beer, some use a carbohydrate mash made of sugar from beet or cane molasses or liquid rice; glucose from corn is popular, too. Others use specially treated millet seeds, kept for a week at the optimum breeding temperature of 90°F. The enzymes that live secrete what becomes riboflavin.

Whatever alchemy of temperature and nutrients produces the most massive reproduction of these little critters becomes the recipe at that particular factory. And it might take five or ten years to find and develop the best strain of bacteria, using genetic modification. But when done correctly, this signature combination could mean patents and big profits. And so it is seemingly worth it, and all, of course, a big secret.

The largest vitamin B2 manufacturer in the world is Guangji Pharmaceutical Co., located in a modern, well-landscaped plant in Hubei, China, on the Yangtze River. While the plant also makes other raw materials for pharmaceuticals and animal feed, it makes over two thousand tons a year of riboflavin, worth more than a billion dollars. Guangji ferments its brew in tanks that can hold ten thousand gallons, and stand as much as six stories high. Expertise in fermentation is common in Asia, thanks to centuries of fermenting rice for wine and soybeans for tofu. The enzymes work for a few days, finally excreting riboflavin.

The vitamin is extracted from the fermentation broth through a complex process that involves multiple steps (concentration, purification, crystallization, drying, and milling) in order to obtain a deep orange flour-like powder that smells slightly stinky (like rotten wood) and is then packed into little twenty-kilogram drums for shipment around the world. The color is due simply to its molecular structure. (Riboflavin is also used as a natural yellow food colorant, often for Easter eggs. If you take extra vitamin B2 supplements your urine turns bright yellow; Guangji had to build a treatment plant just to get rid of the orange in its wastewater).

Without riboflavin, we'd have trouble growing. We'd suffer cracks around the mouth, sores around the nose and ears, a sore tongue, and light-sensitive eyes, and, most important, we would fail to convert food into energy—more than enough reason to include it in the fortification mix.

Folic Acid (B9): The New One

Only a Brit could have discovered folate. In the 1930s, Dr. Lucy Wills found she could cure a certain kind of anemia with Marmite, the dark, yeast-based goo that Brits and Aussies insist on spreading on their morning toast, despite it tasting like a salty, bitter, awful form of molasses. A decade later, the compound was isolated from spinach and named after the Latin word for foliage, *folium* (it is also found in liver, citrus fruits, nuts, and beans, but much of it is destroyed by cooking). Folic acid is the synthetic form for the natural vitamin B9 (folate). Contrary to what you might expect, it is much better absorbed in the synthetic, rather than in the natural form, so if you need to supplement, buy a jar of pills (and don't tell Popeye).

Because it took decades to identify the benefits of folic acid,[4] it wasn't until 1993 that the FDA proposed adding it to the flour enrichment mix, establishing 1998 as the compliance date. But since there was such overwhelming evidence that it could dramatically cut neural tube defects in newborns—as much as 50 to 70 percent—millers went ahead and put it in flour even before labels could be printed, and the FDA was happy to allow it.

Despite its thoroughly Western origins and demand, folic acid, too, comes from China. The modern but modest offices of Niutang Chemical Inc., are based in Changzhou, China, a two-hour drive from Shanghai. A major manufacturer of folic acid as well as the artificial sweetener aspartame, Niutang uses one of the few vitamin-manufacturing processes that is relatively clean and straightforward.

Though they keep the actual technique under wraps, the manufacturers admit that they make B9 with fermented as well as petroleum products. The fermentation is done in starch (usually cane

---

4. Folic acid may even contribute to reduced stroke and heart disease.

molasses, but also tapioca starch or cornstarch). The rest is made from a high-tech soup of an amino acid (glutamic acid, the one that turns into MSG when mixed with sodium; ketchup is full of glutamic acid), a foul-smelling, flammable form of acetone (also found in nail polish remover), and pteroic acid, otherwise known by the catchy nickname, 2-amino-4-oxopteridin-5-yl, or sometimes 4-([2-amino-4-hydroxy-6-pteridylmethyl]amino)benzoic acid, a blend of paraffin and butyric acid, both petrochemicals. (Butyric acid, which is sometimes made through fermentation, is also part of Twinkies' artificial butter flavor.) This forms folic acid—pteroyl-L-glutamic acid—that is in turn refined, reduced in acidity, purified with zinc and magnesium salts, crystallized, dried, and sterilized until only a fine, dark powder remains, ready to ship off to the flour mills.

Mixing It Up

Vitamins are extraordinarily concentrated and used in small amounts, but containers full of vitamins and other additives are stacked high in the factories of blending houses. American Ingredients' facility in Kansas City, Kansas, is one of the largest. It has been converted from an old flour mill into a cool (literally), clean, facility with so much stainless steel and tile that parts of it resemble a modern hotel lobby. Bill Olsen, American's Flour Service Manager, and Don Bruno, its Production Team Leader, escort me through the house. We're all connected by headsets as Bruno plays museum guide, complete with narration.

Custom, premixed enrichment blends are made in an aptly named dump station where plastic bag-lined boxes and little kegs called carboys surround a guy who is armed with scoops, a scale, and a screen-covered, four-foot-diameter hole, which is actually the top of a giant sifter/blender sitting on the floor below. After confronting the mystery of their manufacture, it is a relief to see the actual vitamins. The containers carry labels from all over the world—mostly China and India, but also Europe, and in the case of ferrous sulfate, Indianapolis, Indiana. They are all the consistency of, well, extra-fine flour, for mixing with cake flour such as that used in Twinkies.

I touch a sample of riboflavin, a bright, deep yellow-orange powder, and my hand is instantly coated. As I instinctively wipe it on my black jacket, Olsen and Bruno laugh: they are late in telling me that it stains quite badly, which reminds me of the fact that bright vitamins are used as food (as well as jacket) dyes, too. Like riboflavin, folic acid powder is naturally dark yellow, smooth and moist; thiamine mononitrate and niacin are dull white. Ferrous sulfate is light gray with a bluish tinge, just as you'd expect an iron derivative to look.

Blend recipes are posted on computer screens and on the walls of the dump station. A typical recipe might make a five-thousand-pound batch; while a thousand pounds of one vitamin might be dumped in the hopper, only seventy-three pounds of another might be called for (the industrial equivalent of a pinch of salt). Samples are constantly sent to their high-tech quality control lab, where the mix is examined with extraordinarily sensitive tools such as atomic absorption detectors. Plain, finely powdered, white wheat starch is mixed as a neutral filler, and the blend is conveyed to a robotic packing machine that spits out neat boxes that are sent off to the flour mills for blending into Twinkie flour, bread flour, cracker flour, and cereal—wherever enriched flour is used.

HOUSE BLEND

Over at the still-unidentifiable flour mill, down near the high, open bays where the trucks are loaded, Alexander and I meet up with the chlorinated flour and the vitamin mix from Kansas City in the mill's rather compact blending room. A relatively quiet space housing a forest of 1.5-inch hoses emanating from two dozen small, stainless steel boxes, it looks more like a specialty coffee shop than a factory. Each box, with its precise metering equipment and specialized valves, hums gently, and each contains a different enrichment blend for a different kind of flour. I'm fixated, of course, on the one for cake flour, watching intently as the tubes suck the concentrated yellow-orange blend up and blow it onto the flour as it is conveyed through the hoses.

The hoses feed into a screw conveyor that mixes and blends the flour and the new additives to order. Then, the freshly enriched flour drops into pouches aligned on a bucket conveyor leading out to the loading area. The doses are on such a minute level, as befits potent micronutrients, that accuracy is paramount. Samples are constantly tested for the proper enrichment blend in a nearby lab. A few feet away, six-inch-thick, black hoses dangle like tentacles from the ceilings of three-story-high truck and train bays, blasting properly blended flour into the empty trucks and train cars that are pulling in, loading up for the bakeries.

The law requires only twenty-four milligrams of niacin per pound of flour, and that's the biggest dose in the enrichment mix. Ferrous sulfate weighs in next at twenty milligrams per pound, and the others follow in microdoses of 2.9 milligrams of thiamine, 1.8 milligrams of riboflavin, and only 0.7 milligram of folic acid. This all adds up to 49.4 milligrams of enrichment blend per pound of flour, or one ten-thousandth of a pound of enrichment per pound of flour. Obviously, the amount of added micronutrients in Twinkies is substantially less. At the level of parts per million, it is hardly even a "dash."

After all this effort, only one added item, the mineral ferrous sulfate, affects the Twinkies nutrition label, and is listed as only 2 percent of your daily requirement, at that. The mysterious, complex, international effort made to create this mix of such highly processed, technical supplements stands in stark contrast not only to the natural alternative—whole wheat—but to its unprocessed neighbor in the ingredient list, sugar.

To get sugar, all you do is refine a vegetable. Sort of.

CHAPTER 5

-- -- -- -- -- -- -- --

Sugar

Flour may be the first ingredient on the Twinkie label, but a Twinkie would not be a Twinkie were it not just about half sugar.

Sugar is the second ingredient listed on Twinkies' label, but it could easily be the first. In fact, sugar is the first and most prominent ingredient listed on some Twinkie knock-offs, like Mrs. Freshley's® Creme Cakes. And though Twinkies are certainly sweet—many a fan will admit eating them for the sugar fix alone—it isn't there just for sweetness, not by a long shot.

Of course, it's worth noting that the third and fifth ingredients (the fourth is innocent water) are sugars, too: the corn sweeteners corn syrup and high fructose corn syrup, and some others that contribute to the nineteen grams (four and three-quarters teaspoons; the amount and the recipe change periodically) of sugars in each Twinkie.[5]

---

5. In a way, flour is overshadowed by the sugar and sweeteners that follow it on the ingredient list. In the future, sugars may be broken down on the label by sucrose vs sweeteners, much as fats are now labeled. Sophisticated consumers will embrace that change and the cane sugar industry, which is always battling the corn sweetener industry, will love it.

Sugar is so ever-present in our overall diet, that in the United States, we use 7 to 10 million tons of sucrose (table sugar) each year; Twinkies alone consume four thousand tons annually. That's pure sugar crystals we're talking about here—sugar from live plants, not processing plants—not corn syrup sweeteners, which are a whole other chapter. The reason the Twinkie contains so much sugar? It makes the whole cake work.

NOT JUST SWEETNESS

Ironically, providing sweetness is only a minor job for sugar. Especially in high-ratio cakes like Twinkies, where there is as much or more sugar than flour, sugar is a regular workhorse. It carries flavor, provides color, fosters tenderness, creates an even crumb, and retains some moisture in order to improve shelf life, the holy grail of nearly every packaged food. Other so-called sweeteners just don't share sugar's versatility or importance in baked goods. Without a lot of sugar, cake would be bread.

Sugar starts working its magic way before the batter makes it to the oven. It brings air into the shortening, making for a lighter cake, and does so thanks to the physical shape of its crystals, not through chemistry. When shortening and sugar are mixed during the "creaming" stage of any dessert recipe (especially pie crusts and cakes), the irregular surfaces of sugar crystals trap air in small pockets. These pockets expand during baking when the carbon dioxide formed by the leavening inflates them. That's why it is so important to take your time with the creaming step when baking at home. (If you've ever tried to take a shortcut with creaming, you've probably regretted it in the form of a flatter, denser cake.) Good cakes need bubbles.

The same sugar crystals that are essential for cake are shunned for filling. To get a smooth texture, bakers blend either extra-finely ground sugar, such as Domino® Superfine, or liquid sugar, with the oil and shortening to create a more satisfying mouthfeel while avoiding the grittiness that would come with the use of regular sugar.

In the mixing stage, sugar tenderizes the cake by combining with all the protein it can and absorbing water that would otherwise help build protein and its elasticity. That makes cakes the polar opposite of pizza. Imagine the stretching, pounding, and, of course, tossing and spinning to which pizza dough is subjected. It can withstand all that rough handling because it's loaded with protein and won't easily crumble or break down. Twinkies, on the other hand, use cake flour (which is low in protein) and lots of sugar (to suppress even that protein), and start as a liquid batter. There's no tossing that.

Sugar also stabilizes beaten egg foam, though there is hardly any egg foam found in Twinkies (unlike a true sponge cake, which is made with lots of it). What little there is mixes with the sugar, helping to hold it together until it is baked into its final, familiar, fingerlike form. And yes, that's right, urban legend be damned: Twinkies *are* baked, for a good nine to twelve minutes, at about 350°F, just as you would bake small cakes at home.

Water gets absorbed during baking, too. When the starches heat up, they absorb liquid and swell (called gelatinization by the pros) and eventually solidify, "setting" the cake. As in the mixing stage, sugar competes with starch for the liquid, slowing down its solidification. This also delays the point at which the batter turns into cake, so that the leavening has more time to create gas. Talk about essential teamwork: this is where the fine, uniform grain of a soft, smooth cake crumb is born.

As if that weren't enough, it's at this point in the baking process that sugar helps turn the exposed surface of the cake brown by caramelizing when it reaches over 300°F, giving off more of a welcome flavor and that familiar sweet, baked aroma.

Browned surfaces not only taste good, smell good, and look appetizing, they retain a bit more moisture than the crumb because of their relative denseness. Because Twinkies lack the thick crust of, say, a peasant bread (luckily), every little bit helps to extend their shelf life. Finally, sugar steals water from bacterial cells, further preventing spoilage, which is why sugar is such a well-known preservative. Just think of jams, jellies, all kinds of "preserves" made with sugar, or of containers of honey that last for years. Sugar helps preserve Twinkies, especially the creme filling, in the same way it preserves blueberries.

Multitalented sugar tenderizes and improves the appearance of canned fruit, delays discoloration on the surface of frozen fruits, and enhances flavors in all kinds of desserts, especially ice cream. Even milk can be smoothed and preserved a bit with sugar, as in Eagle Brand® Sweetened Condensed Milk. Sugar balances sour, bitter, and hot flavors in spicy dishes; balances acidic foods like tomatoes and vinegar or sour, bitter tastes in rubs and brines; enhances mouthfeel in drinks and sauces; and strengthens fiber in fruits and vegetables during cooking. Sugar makes dry baked goods like cookies crisp. Of course, let's not forget that sugar's sweet taste is ultimately what drives its popularity. Making foods palatable is what it does in nature as well as in Twinkies. We're hardwired to like sweet foods.

Besides all of these impressive functions, sugar and its derivatives also have some surprising industrial uses: as a flame retardant and plasticizer in polyurethane foam, as a water-based ink for printing on plastic bags, for curing tobacco (spread on leaves to help them dry evenly), and, my personal favorite, for cleaning out cement mixers. Third world medics often use sugar to soak up moisture in wounds that might otherwise grow bacteria. Sugar burns, and can be substituted for charcoal in gunpowder mixtures or mixed with saltpeter to make a cheap smoke bomb. Sugar even

helps fortify cement by hanging on to moisture that would otherwise migrate to the surface and evaporate, a process that delays
setting and makes the cement stronger—which may also explain
some pretty bad cakes I've had.

Sugar Plants

Thinking about where sugar comes from conjures up images
of hot, lush, tropical lands for most of us—it is grown in about
eighty tropical and subtropical countries around the world,
mostly where people like to vacation—but about one-half of refined sugar consumed in the United States (depending on the
year) is made from sugar beets grown in northern climes. Any
green plant can create sucrose from sunlight, air, and water, but
sugarcane and sugar beets do it best. It's all sucrose, pure and
simple. More than 99 percent pure, it so happens.

Hello, Columbus

For most Americans, sugar means Florida. But that's not the
whole story. Sugarcane is a tropical or subtropical grass that
grows as much as twenty feet high; and it's true that our domestic
cane—70 percent of our supply—is grown mostly in Florida, in
the semiartificial, heavily irrigated and engineered, million-acre
Everglades Agricultural Area just south of Lake Okeechobee and
north of the Everglades proper. Some is also grown in Texas and
Louisiana. Since we embargoed Communist Cuba, we import the
most from the Dominican Republic. Worldwide, Brazil is the
biggest producer, followed closely by India.

Caribbean and South American countries have been sending
sugar to Europe for centuries, which is one reason that the French,

Spanish, and British fought over them so often. There may have been more than three thousand sugar mills in the New World prior to 1550, an astounding development that created demand for the equipment that some say triggered the industrial revolution of the 1600s and spurred colonization of our hemisphere. But these mills were not the first. Sugarcane was grown in the South Pacific as many as eight thousand years ago, and it was first refined in India as long ago as 500 BC ("sugar" is derived from Sanskrit for gravel, *sharkara*). Ironically, cane is not even native to the islands. It was introduced to the Caribbean by none other than Christopher Columbus, in 1493, and it has flourished there, dramatically, ever since.

Cane harvesting remains fairly traditional and labor-intensive in the tropics, and people still wade into the thick fields to cut stalks with machetes (after a controlled burn to remove the dried lower leaves). On a sunny vacation beach in Jamaica, a visitor might be shocked to see a billowing cloud of smoke rising across the bay. "No problem, mon—they just burning off the leaves and scaring away the snakes," is the casual and common explanation for what looks like a raging forest fire. Cane's tough, and moist stalks easily survive the fires with no problem, as they say. But since 1992, all sugarcane in Florida is harvested mechanically by large combines, the annual use of guest workers having proved politically difficult. (The big companies still bring in a couple thousand workers each season. And despite all the modernization, they still burn the fields first, taking only fifteen to twenty minutes to burn a forty-acre field).

The harvest unfolds from mid-October to early April because of the immense volume; during this time, cane is cut by specially designed combines that can work in the wet, "muck soil" without sinking. Each combine—smaller but no less expensive and computer-laden than the combines made for harvesting corn and soybeans—replaces sixty hand-cutters, working in large, perfectly rectangular, flat tracts of cane ruled off by a network of straight canals and irrigation ditches and bordered by paved roads. Florida Crystals Corporation of Palm Beach, which harvests about 40 percent of the Florida crop—6 billion pounds a year—processes most of the cane into raw sugar at its largest mill, in Okeelanta, Florida, in the center of cane country, just south of Lake Okeechobee and just west of Palm Beach.

In Okeelanta, as in processing plants near cane fields the world over, the stalks are washed, shredded, and crushed in hot water that dissolves the sugar in order to produce cane juice (the remains of the stalks are dried and burned for fuel—many sugar processors are energy self-sufficient). Impurities are removed by adding lime (calcium hydroxide) and a coagulent to remove them and the lime by turning them into a woolly mass that settles to the bottom. The juice is filtered and evaporated into a syrup through a series of vacuum pans whose low pressure causes the syrup to boil at a low enough temperature to avoid burning and caramelization, a neat trick that was developed by a New Orleans–based engineer named Norbert Rillieux in the 1840s. It revolutionized the industry, and this way of using individual but linked boiling vessels, vacuum pans called effects, to evaporate and crystallize sugar is now used to make many similar food products, including the lactic acid, sodium carbonate, salt, and dairy whey for Twinkies.

Crystals that are 97 to 99 percent sucrose, now labeled raw sugar (which is edible, but a bit dark, because it still contains molasses), are centrifuged out. Rivers of it are hosed into waiting railcars or ocean-going barges, most of which take the sugar up north to places like Domino® Sugar's[6] 1930s-era brick refinery in Yonkers, New York, just north of New York City, for refining and

---

6. Now American Sugar Refining Inc., of which Florida Crystals is part owner.

shipping to regional bakeries, such as the one that makes Twinkies in Wayne, New Jersey. Other ships go to Domino's early 1900s plant on downtown Baltimore harbor, an eleven-story brown brick-and-glass cube that boasts the company's trademark yellow neon sign. The rest of the sugar is refined in Florida.

Kevin McElvaney works for Domino, out of Yonkers, and explains that in days past, the sugar might have gone to Domino's famous 1857 Brooklyn, New York, plant, which is now part of history despite the enormous neon sign that remains atop it. (North American sugar refining started in New York City back in 1799; by 1907, 98 percent of the United States' sugar was refined there, which is when the government busted the New York–based Sugar Trust.) The process of refining sugar is not simple, and the refineries are not small. Some plants refine more than 6 million pounds of sugar a day, though the Yonkers plant, despite being more than a mile long, probably averages no more than around 4 million pounds daily.

Sugar refining (to remove the molasses) continues in much the same way as the original cane processing, according to McElvaney. The raw sugar is dissolved in water to remove impurities and forms a molasses-rich sugar syrup that must be boiled down to crystals in vacuum pans once again, after which the crystals are washed and the molasses centrifuged out, tumbled in rotary driers, screened for crystal size, and then conditioned by blowing humidity-controlled air through them for a few days, readying them for the bulk shipment to the bakeries. Because sugar is heavy and trucking expensive, it is only shipped to bakeries within the refinery's region (New England, mid-Atlantic, mid-South, etc.).

Only a month before, this refined sweetener was still grass, rooted and growing in Florida. That means that while the New York–area Twinkies bakery might get its sugar from Florida via Yonkers, one in Illinois might get its sugar from a decidedly nontropical source, a sugar beet refinery up in Minnesota. Aside from price, there's no discernible difference.

Prussian Cossettes

A sugar beet—a short, rotund root that resembles a turnip—looks totally different from sugarcane, a tall, slender, hard stalk. Think of them as the Laurel and Hardy of sugar. But despite their physical differences, the sugar is separated from the plant in the same way. Unlike most sugarcane, beets are often refined close to the farm, in plants made up of mostly square, steel buildings the size of small stadiums, surrounded by silos. Much is done by co-operatives like Edina, Minnesota–based United Sugar, whose Director of Marketing, Steve Hines, points out that its five plants are in just two states that form the U.S. "Sugar Bowl": North Dakota and Minnesota. United Sugar is the largest sugar marketing organization in the United States, handling more than 5 billion pounds of refined sugar a year, more than 30 percent of the country's total demand. Hines must like snow, because in a neat contrast to the tropical climes where cane grows, nature provides a handy deep freeze for stockpiled beets in the form of long, cold winters.

A Prussian chemist, Andreas Marggraf, first extracted sugar from beets in 1747; beet processing soon became common by the early 1800s. First floated in a flume to wash off rocks, mud, and sand, the beets are then cut into strips, charmingly called cossettes, which look like shoestring potatoes. As with sugarcane, a hot water bath draws the sugar out, forming a sweet juice (the remaining pulp is processed into animal feed). Lime is used here, too, to purify the raw juice, which is then bubbled with carbon dioxide gas to remove the lime and balance the acidity. Next, the sweet juice is boiled under vacuum (to avoid caramelization) until it becomes a syrup. When tiny sugar crystals are dropped into the syrup, to seed it, regular crystals pop up. Molasses is spun off in a centrifuge, leaving pure white crystals ready for use by bakeries.

✳

The Twinkie bakery is probably using the same sugar, with the same extrafine crystals that you buy at the grocery store, but it buys it by the truckload or 100-ton railcar-load. It's then unloaded by either being dropped into a hopper under the car or by being sucked out with fat pneumatic hoses. The bakery conveys it to climate-controlled silos—some of which hold as much as 200,000 pounds—and augurs it over to the bakery in an enclosed (and very dry) conveyor.

Liquid sugar for the filling is delivered by tanker truck 45,000 pounds at a time. And then it's mix, mix, mix—or more accurately, cream, cream, cream—until that shortening is smoothed out and the sugar can start working its many wonders, literally from start to finish.

Refined sugar is pure. Refining it is nothing more than purifying a natural food, McElvaney likes to remind me, a process of separation and removal, not transformation. In sweet contrast to the corn sweeteners that compete for our affection, not one molecule is changed.

- - - - - - - - - -

CHAPTER 6

Corn Sweeteners

Maybe the small lighthouse perched on the Mississippi River levee in Clinton, Iowa, looks a little out of place, but what sounds like a Boeing 747 revving its engine for immediate takeoff is what's startling. The screaming, industrial roar of pure muscle comes from what appears to be a small factory working its way down the river, but is, in fact, a four-story-high, rectangular, white steel tugboat maneuvering a football field–size collection of barges through the strong currents, barely missing the bridge pylons.

This is an everyday occurrence along the river in Iowa and Illinois, where tugs and barges bring thousands of tons of corn to the major plants for processing, including one of Archer Daniels Midland's (ADM), which is close to a mile long. It is served by ADM's barges, ADM'S towboat, and ADM's docks. One barge can hold the equivalent of fifty-two trucks; some towboats lash together as many as twenty barges at a time. A group, called a tow, can be a thousand feet long, just 10 percent short of matching the largest ocean liner ever built, the *Queen Mary 2*. Call it a river liner instead, and note that it carries corn, not caviar.

This plant, made up of dozens of buildings, steam plumes

streaming from their stacks and towers, and ringed by railway sidings loaded with freight cars, used to be the Clinton Corn Processing Company, where high fructose corn syrup was first mass-produced in 1967. Most of our food comes from places like this, because most of our food can be traced back to corn, whether to feed cattle or to make sweeteners for foods ranging from ketchup to Twinkies.

In Sydney, on the other side of Iowa, the soil is as good as you can get for growing corn, so loose, soft, and rich in the early spring you can just plunge your hands into it. As such, the land is so valuable that it is farmed right up to the road's edge, much like the vineyards in France. Most corn is grown on family-owned farms, according to central Illinois farmer Leon Corzine, whose family has done just that for six generations.

Thanks to science and technology, Corzine's generation farms far more efficiently than generations past. Modern farming techniques, including specialized fertilizers, pesticides, and high-tech combines, not to mention doing less versus more (like leaving the "trash" of stems and leaves on the surface, and not tilling the soil), are actually enabling farmers to build topsoil after losing it for many years. Corzine, who is active in farm lobbying organizations, thinks that this Midwestern farmland is the most productive land in the world.

No farm is very far from a group of silos. An estimated 80 million acres of cornfields cover about 125,000 square miles in the United States. The all-time record harvest—almost 12 billion bushels—was recorded in 2004.[7] ADM, the world's largest corn processor, handles 9.5 acres' worth of corn every minute, every

---

7. Almost half is grown from genetically modified (GM) seeds, created by companies like Monsanto to resist its Roundup® herbicide; the trend, thanks in part to Monsanto's strong marketing skills, indicates that there will be more GM corn in the future.

day. Most goes to feed animals, but with as many as six hundred products derived from corn and used in products ranging from auto fuel to pharmaceuticals, plastic fibers to industrial starches (and, lest we forget, sweet drinks and snack cakes), the demand for corn is huge. An astonishing eight of Twinkies' thirty-nine ingredients are made directly from corn—more than from any other single raw material (soybeans are its closest rival, but with only three). If any food symbolizes the almost unimaginably immense corporate agribusiness, corn, the amazing grain, is it.

Nestled in a slight dip in the rolling hills along the Missouri River a few miles southeast of Blair, Nebraska, is a fine example of corporate synergy. There the multinational food giant Cargill (124,000 employees and $71 billion in sales), dubbed the largest privately held company in the United States by *Forbes* magazine (some say the world), has created an industrial campus with a handful of client/partner companies, all of which use something from Cargill's wet-milling corn-processing plant.

Wet Milling on the Missouri

Tall smokestacks spouting clean clouds of water vapor; tank farms; and stark white silos define the skyline. The verticality of these narrow cylindrical forms is offset by boxy, beige, generally nondescript steel buildings. The whole place is surrounded by lines of giant tanker and grain trucks, as well as by black and white tanker railcars on rail sidings. About 175,000 bushels of yellow #2 dent field corn, the national standard commercial crop, arrive at Cargill's plant every day of the year—that's more than 60 million a year—via an endless line of grain trucks, each sporting giant udders of corn waiting to be relieved. The line snakes slowly down a gentle slope from the highway, called the Lewis and Clark

Trail, along the western bank of the Missouri River. A sweet, syrupy smell pervades the air.

Cargill can talk all it wants about the plastics, fuel alcohols, and amino acids that it makes from corn, but the Big Daddy, what brings me to what Cargill calls a biorefinery, is corn syrup, including the ubiquitous high fructose corn syrup that so fascinates my son.

This is no run-of-the-mill mill. It's a complex refinery, and the manager, Eric D. Johnson, is a vice president. After a forty-five-minute PowerPoint presentation in a conference room that would easily hold thirty, we take off on a tour. Every door we encounter in the plant is accessed only by a preauthorized card-key entry. "Industrial espionage" is the explanation offered, and it is why I won't be shown every part of the plant, nor any specialized processing.

Welcome to Blair, Nebraska, a place not known for its gentle climate. Signs pointing to "severe weather shelter" areas are posted in most stairways. Rooftop pipes, insulated and jacketed with sheet metal, are totally pockmarked with deep craters made by hailstones. It's no wonder that one of the buildings on Main Street houses a construction company whose oversize rooftop sign proclaims it a "hail damage specialist." Local car dealerships often lose entire inventories to hail. Luckily, it is a sunny day when I visit.

The first tanks the corn hits after being unloaded, the "steep" tanks, are so massive that you sense rather than see them, like the walls of a skyscraper when viewed from the sidewalk. Climbing harnesses hang by nearby ladders. Each tank, about seven stories high, holds about forty thousand bushels of corn, hot water, and a bit of 0.1 percent solution sulfur dioxide—and there is a gymnasium-size roomful of them. The corn soaks here for a day or two in order to weaken the protein, so that it releases the starch when the kernel gets milled. Amazingly, the steep water is not a waste product but is so nutrient-rich that it becomes a fermentation base for chemicals such as citric acid and amino acids, medicines such as penicillin, and a source of animal feed products.

The loudest room, on a higher floor, is a loft full of motors atop milling vessels—plain, squat, covered vats the size of trucks, where the newly softened corn kernels are wet-milled, or ground up, then physically separated into germ (for oil), fiber (for animal feed), and a gluten/starch mixture, which is then separated by bronze-colored, high-speed centrifuges. Gluten is spun off to become yet another kind of animal feed (chicken or pet food; the yellow corn pigments are what make chickens and yolks yellow), while the liquid starch, the whole point of this operation, is piped up to another level to be washed (up to fourteen times!) and, eventually, refined into all those wondrous corn syrups. (If this was a starch plant instead of a sweetener plant, it would be sent off to be dried, chemically processed, or roasted into various cornstarches. But that's another chapter.)

A sample of fresh, milky cornstarch pulled from a tap on a massive pipe tastes, surprisingly, not sweet at all but bland and sticky. This is the great source of sweeteners, the backbone of the soft drink industry? Hard to believe. But, alas, it's not a sweetener yet.

DIVIDE AND SWEETEN

The path that brought us to this modern biorefinery, to the cutting edge of biology and chemistry and food science, to cheap and versatile sweeteners for modern soft drinks and Twinkies, began centuries ago. Reports of converting Japanese arrowroot starch to sugar date to AD 800, but the current process really began in czarist Russia. In 1811, a chemist by the name of G. S. C. Kirchoff discovered that acid hydrolysis, the process of breaking things down with acid, could be used to produce viscous, sweet syrup by heating potato starch with sulfuric acid. (Legend has it he was chasing Napoleon's offer of a 100,000-franc prize, worth at least about $500,000 today, to anyone who could locate a native sugar source, since France was blockaded and could no longer get West Indian sugarcane—plus, he wanted to create an alternative to British sugar companies. European sugar beets are still a major, and majorly subsidized, crop, and the sugar-producing tropics remain poor, thanks to Napoleon.)

Later, World War I and World War II both caused sugar shortages and thus inspired the North American corn sweetener industry to try harder to find alternatives to cane and beet sugar. Enter corn.

Corn sweeteners are naturally present in cornstarch, despite the fact that it is a thick liquid that's not at all sweet. The key is to separate the sweeteners out. When your body digests a carbohydrate, it breaks it down and absorbs the glucose (also known as blood sugar) for energy. Both your body and the corn sweetener companies do this with enzymes and hydrochloric acid—the same kinds, actually. But while your glands and organs regulate the process in your body, out in Nebraska or Illinois or Iowa, the guys in the control room are in charge.

Put a piece of bread or a cracker on your tongue for a moment and feel it dissolve. Now substitute a seven-story-high steel vat for your mouth and thirteen computer monitors complete with colorized schematics for your glands, and you have a corn syrup plant. We are all miniature Cargills and ADMs, pulling sugar out of potatoes and corn and wheat, which is why white bread is prohibited by the South Beach Diet.

Sucking on bread is not the kind of process one normally associates with high-tech plants, as it seems so, well, natural a process. But, in fact, Americans have been making corn syrup with enzymes instead of acid since the post–Civil War development boom (Union Sugar Company started making corn syrup in New

York in 1865). The first refined version was made in 1866. Since 1967, we've been using enzymes to great effect, as they are very, very accurate and controllable, a big improvement over acid hydrolysis, which often generates unpredictable colors and flavors and is difficult to control.

Breaking Up Is . . . Easy to Do

People in the sweetener industry are totally consumed with the concept of breaking down starch into sugars. When the nice lady at the 800 number of a megacompany that makes corn sweeteners is asked what they do there, she jumps into a long and enthusiastic riff about how starch molecules are very, very long and their job is to cut them up for use in various products, including corn syrups that can be found in Twinkies and soft drinks. Johnson, the manager of the Cargill plant, had likewise welcomed me earlier by saying, "Starch molecules are very, very long, and we break them up here." Later, as we hustle up and down steel ladders surrounding the dozens of huge tanks, he hollers over the industrial hum, "Starch molecules are very, very long, while dextrose molecules are very short, about one-thousandth as long. Enzymes break up those long chains by eating them."

In the nearby quality control lab, a room filled with hundreds of sample bottles and very expensive-looking microscopes and computer equipment, scientists from an enzyme company start with the now-familiar line, "Starch molecules are very, very long . . ." but offer to take the explanation one step further with a great metaphor: starch molecules make up a long train; the enzymes uncouple the cars. Different enzymes and different timing uncouple different quantities of cars, forming different syrups. Break up only a few long sections of the train with the enzyme alpha amylase (the same as in your saliva) and you get just plain corn syrup, thick with its big molecules. Break up more of the train with glucose amylase, de-linking most of the molecules down to the smallest (glucose), and you get dextrose, also called glucose. Rearrange the dextrose train cars via a third enzyme, glucose isomerase, and, bingo, you get high fructose corn syrup.

Enzymes are bred or genetically modified to be so effective that, just as in nature, they can be specifically selected to engineer foods with different mouthfeels or tastes (think cheese). These enzymes trace their genes to a natural microorganism harvested from soil or, in some cases, beef liver. High-tech companies breed them, harvesting them from fungi or bacteria fed by corn and soybean processing by-products. The scientists hand over a bottled sample to me, but it is just muddy water to my untrained eye.

Enzymes are a popular ingredient in detergents (where they break down food stains), gentle drain openers, pulp and paper-making, and, of course, beer-brewing and cheese-making. They are helpful in textiles, too, having replaced pumice stone for "stonewashing" blue jeans, among other "finishing" tasks. And they are essential for making Twinkies, used to extract four different sweeteners from cornstarch: plain corn syrup, dextrose crystals, glucose syrup, and, above all, high fructose corn syrup.

And none of this bears any resemblance to your home cooking.

- - - - - - - - - -

CHAPTER 7

Corn Syrup, Dextrose, Glucose, and High Fructose Corn Syrup

The corn syrup plants remind me of a good restaurant buffet, complete with dishes that would be satisfying on their own, but create a banquet when assembled as a meal. The wet milling industry offers a whole range of finished products, each of which stands on its own, but taken together make for great cakes.

CORN CANDY AND MORE

The first Twinkie ingredient made from cornstarch is simple corn syrup, the same as that clear, Karo® Light corn syrup you probably have on your pantry shelf. It's the only corn syrup product in Twinkies for which there is a home version.

The big plants make it in a couple different ways. Either the liquid starch is put into a vat the size of a small house along with hydrochloric acid (for the acid hydrolysis process), or else the starch gets mixed with the enzyme alpha amylase and maybe a little lime or caustic soda (to adjust the pH), after which it's heated just a bit and left for a few hours to convert into 25 percent dextrose, which is then ready for processing into other syrups and dextrin. Another pH adjustment stops the enzyme activity, and voilà, corn syrup.

Corn syrup's viscosity, a product of the remaining long molecules that were not "chopped up" by the enzymes or acid, makes it useful as, well, a thickener. It is often used somewhat like dry cornstarch. In fact, maltodextrin, a stronger thickener that is usually dried and powdered, but which works more like the starches described in the next chapter, is created at this point by cooking the cornstarch solution just a bit less than needed to make corn syrup. Like any thickener, maltodextrin can be used as a fat replacer; the ingredient label on Smucker's® Reduced Fat Natural Style Peanut Butter even says specifically, "(replaces fat)."

Corn syrup is only about a third as sweet as table sugar, so it is only partly used as a sweetener (and is often paired with another in desserts). Industrial bakers rely on it for its ability to stabilize and soak up moisture in a way that allows them to keep water to a minimum while baking a moist cake, thus preventing spoilage, and it does this without adding intense sweetness in the way that sugar or honey does. Corn syrup helps with the browning, too (substitute some corn syrup for sugar in your cookies if you want them browner). Not only does corn syrup not crystallize like cane sugar, it actually prevents crystallization, which is why it's so popular in candy (it's usually the main ingredient in the cheap stuff), ice cream, and frozen desserts. It's the main ingredient in Marshmallow Fluff® and lasts six to twelve months without refrigeration. These days, you can hardly find a sweet food that doesn't contain corn syrup—even home recipes call for it.

Most corn syrup that doesn't find its way into baked goods goes into dessert foods such as fruit fillings, frostings, cookies, as well as vitamins (as a filler, often in the form of glucose), and into beer as a yeast food for fermentation. It even helps suspend the mix of ingredients in salad dressings (it's the second ingredient, right after water, in Kraft® Free French Style Fat-Free Dressing), condiments, and that old favorite dessert food, hot dogs.

Dextrose Is Not Always Dextrose

While corn syrup is familiar to home cooks, dextrose is certainly not. A second enzyme reaction in another room-size vat goes on for as many as seventy-two hours, concentrating the starch into what is called a pure dextrose solution, about 98 percent dextrose. There's a small, three-way fork in the stream at this point, when some of this dextrose is pumped to another part of the plant to be made into high fructose corn syrup, some is pumped out of the plant to serve as a feedstock for its neighbors making industrial products, and some becomes the dextrose and glucose found in Twinkies.

This dextrose solution is popular stuff. One of the neighbors on the Blair campus ferments it into lactic acid for sodium stearoyl lactylate, also a key emulsifying ingredient in Twinkies. Some of the others there and at other wet milling plants ferment the dextrose into alcohol (especially ethyl alcohol, or ethanol, for fuel, alcoholic beverages, or industrial use), amino acids (including glutamate, for making monosodium glutamate [MSG]), citric acid, xanthan gum (a thickener), or even plastic. Dextrose is the fermentation base for vitamin C, as well as penicillin and other antibiotics. Some goes on to be hydrogenated into sorbitol and made into the popular emulsifier polysorbate 60. Simply calling corn syrups "sweeteners" seems to be doing them an injustice.

The crystallized dextrose listed on Twinkies' labels is a bulking agent—an ingredient that adds fewer calories than the ingredient it replaces—that is also beloved, along with its other corn sweetener cousins, for its ability to cause browning through the Maillard reactions (when sugars and proteins react under heat).

y adds some brown color and smooth texture to
rusts when they are baked, which may be why it also
Doritos Nacho Cheese®. Dextrose crystals provide a
cool feel and a desirable sheen to a filling like that in Twinkies
without adding too much sweetness (corn-derived dextrose is
only about 60 to 70 percent as sweet as table sugar), similar to
what it does in ice cream and frozen desserts. It is completely fer-
mentable (whereas cane sugar is not) so it serves as a successful
yeast food in bread and beer. It preserves as well as cane sugar but
doesn't obliterate the taste of fruit in candies, jams, jellies, carbonated beverages, and even preserved meats. Dextrose is second
only to sugar in marshmallows, and is the first ingredient in
Kraft® Sure-Jell Premium Fruit Pectin for Homemade Jams & Jellies, offering "25% less sugar than regular pectin." High-stress
athletes know dextrose can be taken directly to boost their blood
sugar levels quickly—but that also means it is used in pharmaceuticals and other products for which delivering energy to the
bloodstream quickly is paramount.

You can buy European dextrose in grocery stores, either a
granular or an ultrafine white powder, confusingly labeled as glucose (the traditional name for it). And if that weren't confusing
enough, actual glucose only makes things more complicated.

SYRUP AND SHOE POLISH

One of the more curious aspects of this highly organized,
science-based industry is that the pros—at major companies' tech
support call centers, on their various Web sites, in their various
catalogs, or in response to various inquiries—do not agree on the
meaning of the term "glucose" as listed on Twinkies' labels. I've
deduced that Hostess probably puts two names for the same
thing on the ingredient list because the FDA requires the listing of

"the most commonly used name" for each ingredient, regardless of technical duplication (same molecule, different form—kind of like ice and water). Essentially, regardless of what they're called, these sugars do basically the same thing.

In Twinkies' crumb and filling, glucose syrup, like dextrose powder, is used to add bulk and sweetness and to help in browning, but its main job is retaining moisture so the cakes don't dry out. Glucose syrup rounds out the texture and flavor of cough syrups and lozenges and also helps enhance the flavor of prepared meats.

Glucose does basically the same thing—acts as a terrific humectant—in a lot of nonfood products, too: it adds smoothness, flavor, and shelf life to tobacco; brings glossiness and pliability to shoe leather; stabilizes adhesives; prolongs the setting of concrete; moisturizes air fresheners; and controls evaporation of perfumes. It helps hand lotion stay moist on your shelf for years—essentially acting as a moisturizer for a moisturizer.

However, despite the obvious benefits to shining shoes and softening faces, dextrose and glucose are not the big draw here. The main attraction is high fructose corn syrup, and that dextrose solution being piped around the plant has a real date with destiny.

How Sweet Is It?

It's time to find my son some answers. High fructose corn syrup (HFCS) is a veritable Zelig of a food ingredient, found in food products of all kinds. In the lobby of the Blair plant stands a display showcasing some of its clients' wares—all well-known, nationally distributed, processed foods that shall remain unnamed at Cargill's request—fruit, sports, and soft drinks galore, of course, along with wine coolers, yogurts, breads, cereals, meats, sauces, condiments, even pet food, and, of course, the inevitable cakes. The gamut represents the epitome of popular processed foods.

Their makers prefer the stability, reliable supply, easy mixing, and of course, the low price of this alternative to sugar.

HFCS is an ingredient that has literally changed consumer product icons: taste a common, major-brand soft drink like a cola or iced tea abroad, where it may still be sweetened with sugar instead of HFCS, and you might be startled at the difference. Many people find the sugar-sweetened drink is cleaner and crisper-tasting, and perhaps more thirst-quenching due to its lack of aftertaste. In Twinkies, high fructose corn syrup works with its less-sweet but much thicker cousin, plain corn syrup, to perform a variety of important functions: give body to both the cake and the filling; give color to the cake through browning (via the Maillard reactions); soak up moisture and control microbiological growth; and, of course, sweeten the whole thing without the risk of crystallization that regular sugar presents. Leave some simple sugar syrup out for a few days and crystals will form on the sides and bottom of the container; not so with HFCS. For the manufacturers of packaged foods like Twinkies, HFCS is no mere sugar substitute—it is, in fact, a huge improvement.

For the consumer, cheap, plentiful HFCS is decidedly a mixed blessing—some love the fact that its cost-effectiveness and ubiquity means that more sweet foods are available, while others decry its infiltration into our food chain and link it directly to the dramatic increase in obesity and diabetes. The debate about its merits and problems rages daily, much to the industry associations' consternation. The industry mostly assigns the blame for the country's problems with obesity to a lack of exercise, or cites the fact that you can't link these issues directly with high fructose corn syrup because sugar consumption has actually dropped proportionately with the increase in the consumption of HFCS. The Corn Refiners Association, for example, insists, in a booklet entitled *Corn: Part of a Healthy Diet*, that HFCS and table sugar (sucrose) are metabolized in exactly the same way once they are absorbed into the bloodstream. Industry Web sites state that Mexicans and Europeans are experiencing rising rates of obesity and diabetes while consuming far less HFCS than we do, and industry press releases state that studies concluding the contrary are flawed (some critical studies did indeed deal only with fructose, not a blend of fructose and glucose such as HFCS or table sugar). In fact, the industry's position, that problems linked with HFCS may have more to do with larger portion sizes, is easy to accept. People are simply eating way more processed food, which also happens to contain HFCS. (Of course, the industry advertises to encourage such consumption, but that's the American way.) The food and agriculture industry educational group, International Food Information Council (IFIC), points out that while 600 more calories per person per day are "available" now that weren't back before HFCS became commonly used (1980), HFCS and sucrose account for only about 10 percent of the added calories we are consuming. Meanwhile, it seems that soft drinks containing HFCS have an awful lot to do with this—but mostly because of their size, not because of their sweetener. In the 1950s, soda was sold in 6.5- or 8-ounce bottles (containing 88 to 100 calories per serving) as an occasional refreshment; today, it is regularly served in 20-ounce bottles (at 240 calories a pop) and sometimes even 64-ounce servings (what does Coca-Cola expect you to put into its Monster Mug—milk?). More important, today, soft drinks are far more often consumed as a common, mealtime beverage, than as a special treat.

Ultimately, most experts agree that we Americans (and those in modernized cultures elsewhere) eat too much low-fiber, refined food. Ask a nutritionist if HFCS is OK for you, and he or she will probably tell you to exercise more and to eat fewer calories, more whole grains and minimally processed food, especially fruits and vegetables, kind of sidestepping the HFCS controversy but also—pointedly or inadvertently, it's not clear—encouraging the avoidance of HFCS itself. But many scientists and consumers, concerned that HFCS adversely affects things like our trigylceride and insulin levels, leading to type 2 diabetes and obesity, would not be satisfied with that answer. Dr. Richard Anderson, a research chemist at the USDA's Beltsville Human Nutrition Research Center, considers HFCS a "huge problem," because it is metabolized differently than other sugars, directly contradicting the industry line. He further confirms, "I would definitely make the link [to obesity and diabetes] with the increase in the intake of fructose." As straightforward as that statement seems, however, it's not conclusive, because HFCS and cane sugar have roughly the same amount of fructose.

Scientists know where to look (the liver and the pancreas, for starters) but here in the early 2000s, after thirty years of common use, the proper broad and long-term studies about the effects of HFCS still aren't being done. This leaves a big knowledge gap into which emotion and politics easily flow. The question is central not only to our national health policies but to our billion-dollar agricultural-industrial policies (corn farming is heavily subsidized; a lot of the complaints about HFCS come from subsidy-loving, sugar-growing states). It is clearly an unresolved issue from the consumer's health's point of view. Both sides agree that more and better studies are needed. And unless it is found that HFCS truly interferes with your pancreas and liver, and unless consumers and their government turn their backs on artificial sweeteners, biorefineries like the one in Blair will keep cranking out high fructose corn syrup by the ton.

＊

The air in the plant smells syrupy sweet, but since the actual processing area is off-limits to visitors, I can't identify the source. Obviously, each company competes intensely to find the most efficient conversion process in this expensive undertaking, so precise details are not offered by anyone. Most follow a highly technical process called isomerization that was developed around 1970, where the pure dextrose gets pumped through a several-story-high tower that is filled with little beads containing an extremely efficient and precisely targeted enzyme, glucose isomerase. Each time the dextrose passes through the tower, molecules are actually rearranged, and some of the glucose changes into fructose, resulting in a higher concentration of fructose, and a sweeter syrup. Putting the same atoms in different positions allows the engineers to produce syrups of varying degrees of sweetness for different customers' needs.

Even though the tower might hold tens of thousands of gallons, each pass-through takes only a matter of minutes. Then it goes through another set of similar towers called fractionation units, where the glucose and fructose are separated, purified, and recombined, mixing and remixing what was already sliced and diced. Although 42 percent high fructose syrup is common and typically used in Twinkies (and most cakes), 55 percent high fructose corn syrup is the big deal, the one used in most popular soft drinks. The remaining percentages—58 percent or 45 percent respectively—of the high fructose corn syrup is glucose that was not converted to fructose, plus a smidgeon of other sugars (table sugar, or sucrose, is a fifty-fifty mixture of fructose and glucose). I can't wait to tell my son: high fructose corn syrup is cornstarch cooked with enzymes. Elementary!

When corn refiners first tried to make sweeter syrup on a major industrial level, they had trouble raising the fructose levels. The first shipment, in 1967, was only 14 percent fructose. The sweetener industry folks got their "high" when they achieved 42 percent in 1968, and then 55 percent in the late 1970s. Such dedication was worth it—the product took off exponentially within only a few years. Since 1980, when it was first used in Coca-Cola®, HFCS has replaced sugar in every major American soft drink. It's come a long way from czarist Russian chemistry. We can at least thank the Russians (or is it Napoleon?) for this invention as we sip our sodas.

✳

Johnson, my host, silently opens a door, smiling knowingly. Steep stairs lead onto steel grating, which hovers over railcars and a tank truck with hoses as thick as my leg draped into the holes at the top. The railcar is being cleaned with 180°F water, but the stainless steel mesh hose going into the tank truck is carrying the mother lode—the ultimate, ubiquitous, freshly made high fructose corn syrup.

In a small office perched on a balcony between two apparently surgically clean bays, a huge, bearded technician, whom I'll call Bruce, appears dressed to perform minor surgery. In white coveralls and a mask, Bruce has just returned from climbing onto the big tank truck to get a sample, and now hovers over a microscope-like tool called a refractometer. A thick yellow climbing harness still dangles from his thighs. "Just checkin' the solids," he drawls. This is a batch of 55 percent high fructose corn syrup, the real McCoy, and this Blair plant, like any other midsize plant, can produce as many as 5 million pounds—that's twenty-five railcars—of high fructose corn syrup each day.

Small sample bottles of the clear liquid are scattered on the desk, begging to be tasted. A slow sip of this much maligned elixir reveals a rather thin syrup without too much pancake syrupy mouthfeel, and an intense sugar rush. "That's as fresh as you can get," Bruce says proudly.

Nebraska's finest. And its thinness stands in marked contrast to the corn thickeners made elsewhere in the Midwest—cornstarch and its siblings.

CHAPTER 8

Corn Thickeners: Cornstarch, Modified Cornstarch, Corn Dextrins, Corn Flour

When a cornstarch company says its products make foods "smoother, creamier, chewier, crunchier, softer, denser, healthier, or lighter," one might be inclined to ask, why not add that they promise instant weight loss, instant wealth, and while we're at it, infinite longevity? If an ingredient like cornstarch can really do all that, you could be excused for feeling that cornstarch and corn flour get too little respect.

Many associate corn flour with simply keeping food (pizza, bread) from sticking to oven bottoms, packages, and baking pans. Cornstarch is famous for such pedestrian tasks as thickening sauces, or for keeping dry mixes dry and flowing. Neither seems to boast a glamorous list of accomplishments. But, in fact, corn flour and cornstarch are multitalented contributors to the food biz and even more popular in the industrial/nonfood world.

Despite being a household staple, cornstarch is used to make way more cardboard than cakes. Only a bit more than 7 percent of the cornstarch made finds its way back into food like Twinkies (out of about 750 million pounds made yearly). A full two-thirds is used to make paper and cardboard. (For detractors of Twinkies or bland food and bad gravies, that statistic may not come as a surprise.) The (roughly) remaining 27 percent is used to make my kids' favorite toy, biodegradable packaging "peanuts," to keep textiles smooth and collars stiff, and to keep baby bottoms dry, all a far cry from food and Twinkies. Looking to the future, it seems likely that many cornstarch products can replace petroleum-based, nonrenewable resource-devouring products, such as biodegradable plastic film, fabrics, carpeting, cups, food containers, and even furniture. The hottest ticket in development is corn-based fabrics for clothing, though it is not clear whether that would be biodegradable, too. One thing is certain: cornstarch's future is not in food.

The cornstarch used in Twinkies is likely to come from specialized wet milling plants that use good old yellow #2 dent field corn and make nothing but starch. While the Cargill plant in Blair concentrates on sweeteners, others, such as the Tate & Lyle plant in Lafayette, Indiana, or the nearby National Starch plant in Indianapolis, concentrate on starches (both firms are members of British global chemical conglomerates). Though National's 125-acre plant is not one of the largest, it ships an impressive 4-plus million pounds of starch a day.

Sweetener and starch plants use pretty much the same process. There's a fork in the road of the flowchart, with slurry for syrups ("sweeteners") veering off to one side and slurry for starches veering off to the other. What's cool is that both forks lead to Twinkies. Dedicated starch plants use a softer type of corn than syrup plants, called waxy maize or waxy corn. This corn was bred for seed during World War II from a 1908 Chinese import, when Southeast Asian supplies of tapioca, the more common source of cooking starch, were cut off. Potatoes, rice, and wheat are also common starch sources that are sometimes blended, which is why food labels often say just "food starch." At a starch plant, this liquid starch is dried, chemically modified, or roasted so there's something for everyone: plain cornstarch, modified cornstarch, and dextrins. (Some plants make more than four hundred different kinds of starches for industrial and food uses for far more products than Twinkies.) But as far as Twinkies are concerned, there are only three kinds of starch.

PLAIN AND SIMPLE

Plain cornstarch, a fine white powder, is what you buy in the supermarket. Since it starts out as a milky soup, the challenge is to dry it. And, since the water cannot be boiled out, nor can the starch be heated too high (because it would swell into a soft, pudding-like mass, similar to what you'd get if you added corn-starch to hot gravy), the starch solution is "dewatered" through massive presses and centrifuges. At National Starches' Indianapolis plant, the moist granules are then conveyed into the bottom of machinery so extraordinary, it calls to mind a sort of techno-Indianapolis answer to the St. Louis Gateway Arch. This is the ring dryer, a bright silver vertical circle with a 150-foot diameter that blasts the starch on a roller-coaster ride in a bed of warm (but not too hot) air and then sends it off to be packed into bags or rail-cars, all without cooking it by mistake.

Food starches have been separated from vegetables since ancient Chinese and Egyptian times (wheat starch was used to make papyrus, cosmetics, and must have helped keep the pleats in the pharaohs' royal outfits, but there was no corn there—corn is an American thing). Refining corn for food use started in the United States with the founding of Thomas Kingsford's eponymous Oswego, New York, firm in 1848. By 1880 it was the largest company of its kind in the world, with a thousand employees making thirty-five tons of cornstarch daily. Kingsford's Starch, originally used primarily for laundry, was (along with baking powder) one of the first truly national consumer products that was advertised extensively, and the firm is credited with revolutionary innovations in corn refining that led right up to today's modern plants. One of the post–World War II accomplishments occurred when drying tables hundreds of yards long were replaced with centrifuges that spun the water out; another was angling the "steep tank" walls so that new corn could be added (on the side) and continuously removed (from the center). These seemingly simple changes allowed for faster, continuous processing with less labor, assuring a low and popular price.

Kingsford's merged with Argo, a Nebraska firm, in 1899, but both brands are still sold today, a testimony to consumer loyalty. The catch is that Kingsford's brand is only found in Philadelphia, southern and northern California (though apparently not in central California), Denver, and, in a considerable leap of logic as well as ocean, Hawaii. You gotta love those marketing guys.

Cornstarch can be found in products as varied as mayonnaise, gumdrops, and chocolate candy fillings. Because it soaks up moisture so well, cornstarch, used dry, keeps confectioners' sugar and packaged cake mixes dry and free-flowing. It works so well in baking powder that it is found in all the major brands, and sets the flavors on the surface of snack foods like Wise® Cheez Doodles®. Used wet, it helps both candy and salad dressings set, extends Cheerios® crispiness in milk, and binds moisture in processed meats like Oscar Mayer® Turkey Bologna.

At home, you can make classic white sauce with it (just cook gently with milk and butter), and make a passable cake flour from all-purpose flour by adding a little cornstarch to it. Mixed with baking soda and water, it makes some fun modeling clay; a little dumped into a tub of warm bathwater soothes irritated skin (a lot dumped in makes for a major plumbing problem).

But because cornstarch tends to form a gel after it is heated, it's a great thickener and texturizer (imparting "body") for moist things that you cook: soups, sauces, gravies, custard, fruit pie fillings, and puddings (cornstarch essentially *is* the pudding in simple recipes, along with sugar, milk, and egg yolks or margarine). Heat some liquefied cornstarch in a bowl by itself and it forms a chunk of gel that stays moist on the inside for days.

Starch helps keep Twinkies' sponge cake springy and prevents crumbling, thus extending its shelf life. And along with modified cornstarch and dextrins, it provides texture (firmness, creaminess, and aeration) as well as moisture control to Twinkies' creamy filling.

A Pockle Now

As anyone who has struggled to make gravy knows, regular cornstarch has to be heated and stirred just so in order to avoid congealing. Since it also doesn't last long—it simply swells and then disintegrates—the big bakeries demand something a little more forgiving, something that doesn't require the loving care and attention of a home cook.

Just after World War II, scientists successfully made starches dramatically more useful, and especially so since 1960, with the cultural push for convenience foods. As a result, the big food processors can order something called a pre-gel, or pregelatinized starch, which has been chemically altered to thicken at various temperatures, including cold ones, and then stay swollen, providing a huge time and handling advantage to industrial bakers. (Unfortunately, no consumer version exists.)

To get starch to do this, though, there's a trade-off. It's put through a chemical bath that one chemical engineer prefaces as "the part you're not going to like." He is right. In the most common process (there are many), regular cornstarch is mixed in reactor vessels that can hold up to sixty thousand gallons (the size of a dozen tank trucks), along with propylene oxide (a petroleum product made from natural gas, chlorine, and lye or hydrochloric acid) and a watery, volatile, pungent liquid called phosphorus oxychloride that is so reactive it is handled as a hazardous material. Made from phosphorus, oxygen, and chlorine (P-O-C), which give it the rather cute nickname of "pockle," it reacts violently with water to make hydrochloric and phosphoric acid and modifies and chlorinates the target molecules. Besides making Twinkie ingredients, pockle makes an unlikely group of products that includes pesticides, pharmaceuticals, and dyestuffs—but, as industry members say, has been used safely in food for fifty years. That may be because it is used here in a strength of less than one-tenth of 1 percent.

Sometimes the starch is bleached or treated with sulfuric or hydrochloric acid specifically to make such things as pie fillings. It takes only a few hours in the reactor vessel, agitated by a spinning propeller, to make this miracle food. The strong chemicals, bleach, and acids are easily washed out before the starch is dried and ready for making dessert.

The resulting liquid is sprayed into giant hot-air tanks, flash-dried to form a white powder that not only helps Twinkies seem denser, but above all, moister. Modified cornstarch is all about texture through moisture control, the home equivalent of expensive and hard-to-handle eggs and cream, which is why it saves food companies big bucks.

While the process may not be, modified starch is easy to swallow and makes drinks extra-smooth, and so finds its way into nutritional beverages for the elderly and the infirm; it provides the all-important gelling ability in instant puddings and Kraft® Jet-Puffed® Marshmallows. It improves the freeze-thaw behavior in microwave meals. And it mimics, with few or no calories, that smooth mouthfeel and tongue-coating that used to be the exclusive domain of fat in low-fat desserts and salad dressings, frustrating dieters who are trying to avoid all processed carbohydrates while eating low-fat foods. It is the primary ingredient in Knorr® instant Hollandaise Sauce Mix, which contains no eggs. That's why it also plays an essential role in forming Twinkies' creamy filling, and it doesn't need any cooking. It locks in water, keeping it from "weeping" into the cake while on the shelf. In short, modified cornstarch helps us cheat, but cheat well.

This unique property is what allows Dave Krishock, baking instructor at the Kansas State University Department of Grain Science and Industry, to describe the stabilized creme filling in this way: "You pump it in and it stays forever."

Drinking and Firefighting Don't Mix

The thick liquid cornstarch flowing from the wet mill gets hit with a double whammy of heat and acid when it is made into dextrins, also called thinned starches, which despite the name tend to be very concentrated. The dextrinizer, which holds ten to twenty thousand pounds of starch powder, heats and mixes the starch with a touch of hydrochloric acid, causing a chemical breakdown that turns it dark, sweet, and, most important, sticky. Later, the starch is dried to a white or yellowish powder, depending on what the mix master wants to make (more often cardboard than cake). Food is a sideshow, here.

Among its many uses, dextrins are responsible for the glossy sheen on printing paper, the glue on postage stamps and envelopes (due to its marvelous ability to remain inert when dry but turn adhesive when wet, and—let us not forget—to not poison us). Much of it is used to provide the glue in paper bags and corrugated cardboard boxes. Still, despite these rather unappetizing uses, it is still a regular food product, just not a good-tasting one.

Using cornstarch as glue was accidentally discovered, the

legend goes, in Dublin in 1821, during the celebration of a visit by King George IV. A fire broke out in a textile factory that used potato starch for finishing cloth. Six workers, drunk on whiskey, fell into the starch water tank while trying to man the fire pump. When they finally got out, they were stuck together, and a new use was found for starch (as well as a new image for teamwork). The official version is far less dramatic, noting only that a worker observed after a fire that this roasted, brown stuff made a thick, adhesive paste when dissolved in water. No matter where the truth lies, in a slap to Irish separatists, it became known as British gums.

Whiskey and Twinkies

Corn flour is the odd man out here. First of all, it is not a thickener like the starches, though it almost works like one. And unlike cornstarches and corn syrups, which are wet-milled, corn flour is dry milled, an older and simpler process with its roots in a popular product quite unlike Twinkies. ADM's giant, Peoria, Illinois, dry-milling plant, which dominates much of the city's Illinois River waterfront, is itself dominated not by its twenty-story grain elevators, web of train-size conveyor belts, or ten-story-high processing towers, but by massive and handsome antique brick buildings that were built during its previous life as a Hiram Walker whiskey distillery. Unfortunately for me, no whiskey odors remain.

Despite its incessant drive to use the latest and greatest technology, and despite calling the process dry milling, industrial corporate dry millers use a technique to soften the outer shells of corn kernels that was developed by Native Americans millennia ago: they give the kernels a quick soak in, or a spray with, a hot water and caustic soda (lye) solution. Whether making tortillas or

Twinkies, it starts the same way. After that, the process for making corn flour resembles wheat flour milling except that a lot of it goes into making food alcohol, usually for whiskey, or nowadays, ethanol, for fuel.

First, rollers crush the kernels so that the germ can be removed for making corn oil. The subsequent series of mills crush the remaining parts into descending levels of coarseness: coarse grits (hominy), flaking grits (for cornflakes and other breakfast cereals), brewers' grits, cornmeal, and, ultimately, fine flour. Various grades of crushed kernels go on to become cattle feed or even diesel fuel (biodiesel) and explosives. Milling for tortillas and real corn chips skips the degerming part—that's why traditional chips have such a nice, crunchy texture. And the brewers mentioned here include more than whiskey makers: they brew beer, antibiotics, industrial enzymes, and even vitamin C with corn grits. Corn is fertile stuff.

Surprisingly, corn flour is an important addition to the wheat flour used in making Twinkies. Not simply relegated to dusting countertops, it provides a unique gel-like texture to the crumb that holds both the structure and the moisture in a little bit and, of course, helps to prolong Twinkies' shelf life.

✳

The whole corn product team is one big moisture-holder and life-extender for Twinkies, but its value extends far beyond cakes and fillings to salad dressings, snack foods, and meat. Simply put, starch is practically an Olympic athlete among food additives. And yet, despite its impressive accomplishments, it can't claim to bring everything to life—that's a job for plain and simple H_2O.

- - - - - - - - - - -

CHAPTER 9

Water

Water is the only ingredient that isn't delivered to the Twinkie bakery by vehicle, and it is the only truly local ingredient at any bakery, yet even *it* is processed. It's one of the few Twinkie ingredients that is used in the exact same form as we use in our homes. But even water's source is traceable and not without intrigue.

New Jersey's Wanaque Reservoir, opened in 1930, supplies more water than any other facility in that populous state: more than 173 million gallons per day. Six and a half million gallons of that travel to Wayne, New Jersey, so there is plenty to supply the big Hostess bakery there that makes Twinkies for most of the Northeast. And it is good, clean water, freshly chlorinated and filtered, delivered straight from the water main by the Wayne Township Department of Public Works.

There are plenty of water treatment options for an end user like a major bakery, including coagulation, disinfection, pH adjustment, ion exchange, membrane filtration, and carbon filtration (especially effective at removing chlorine and fluoride), but in Wayne, New Jersey, very little is required, and whatever, if anything, is done is confidential. All bakeries wrestle with local water quality. For example, sometimes a recipe ends up needing to be modified with a little extra calcium sulfate or flavoring to balance acidity. Whatever it might take in Wayne, it would not be a big challenge to the Twinkie bakery.

NO GOOEY MESS

Bread may be known as the staff of life, but water is what turns flour into bread. Water is essential for life—and water brings life to Twinkies, literally bringing a dry mixture of powders alive. I love that moment of truth in baking, the point of no turning back, when I pour the water into the dry ingredients and start mixing. That's when the action really begins.

The Twinkie, like anything cooked by recipe, is a kind of ecosystem in which each ingredient plays out its role in relation to the others; but water is the one ingredient that ties all them all together. Once the bakery mixes water into the dry ingredients to form a batter, it starts reacting in ways that eventually transform passive powders into active reagents, each with specific roles in numerous chemical reactions to come (the technical term is "baking"). This crucial moment is often just that—two to five minutes in a five-foot-wide "mixing bowl" that stands three and a half feet high (and holds up to two thousand pounds) before the batter is pumped into the continuous mixer, vigorously massaged for ten to twenty seconds, and then squirted into the rapidly moving Twinkie molds that are proceeding, twenty-four hours a day, into the conveyor ovens (at 500 million Twinkies a year, things move quickly).

The liveliest effect occurs when the double-acting baking powder undergoes the first of its two reactions (the second is triggered by the heat of the oven). Water invigorates the proteins in the flour so that gluten begins to form; then, the now-liquefied sugar starts to slow them down, as does the shortening. Water re-activates powdered eggs and dissolves almost all of the other in-gredients to create the texture of the cake. It dissolves or disperses the cornstarches, corn flour, soy protein isolate, cellulose gum, sweet dairy whey, salt, mono and diglycerides, flavors, sodium stearoyl lactylate, sodium and calcium caseinate, calcium sulfate, sorbic acid, Yellow No. 5, and Red No. 40. It triggers the emulsi-fiers, mono and diglycerides, polysorbate 60, and lecithin, to do their work, linking water and oil in both the cake and the filling. The whole mix is transformed, first by water and then by heat, into something that did not exist before.

Just as we cannot live without water, neither could a Twinkie. A Twinkie would be nothing more than an oily, gooey mess with-out it. And much of that oil and goo comes from soybeans.

CHAPTER 10

Soy: Partially Hydrogenated Vegetable and/or Animal Shortening, Soy Lecithin, and Soy Protein Isolate

Giant machines with open maws that could swallow a bear, lips made of rotating spiral blades the length of cars, pointed teeth four times the size of traffic cones, and jagged-edged circular knives surround me, and all I can think is: Martha Stewart would love this.

I suppress both the urge to laugh and the urge to share this rather bizarre association with the farmer showing me the machines, but, I swear, it is not so far-fetched. It's a perfectly logical association I've made—I'm at the world's largest John Deere equipment dealership, in Assumption, Illinois, and the stray soybean seeds left in one of the machines (a planter) are pastel-colored, just like Martha's famed Araucana hens' eggs. These soybeans have been treated with a fungicide and are colored to make the point. They are Monsanto's Roundup Ready® seeds, which grow into soy plants that resist the popular herbicide. Most of the United States' soybean crop is grown from this kind of genetically modified seeds—80 or 90 percent, in fact (Monsanto controls much, if not most, of the seeds in the world). And these plants are the source of one of the essential baking ingredients in Twinkies and every home kitchen: vegetable short-ening.

Soy is one of the most successful and efficient foods in history, and it contributes two other very important ingredients to Twinkies, lecithin and soy protein isolate. Not only is soy full of complete proteins—around 35 percent by weight—but its oil can also be used in such diverse products as anticorrosion agents, diesel fuel, and waterproof cement (presumably very healthy ce-ment). But most of the soybeans grown here—some say as much as 94 percent—are turned into animal feed, not Twinkies.

Despite their dramatic impact on our lives, soybeans, like corn, are a good crop for smaller, not corporate, farms, where they are often grown in equal acreage. Greg Anderson is a fifth genera-tion family farmer, with several hundred acres near Newman Grove, Nebraska, a bit northwest of Omaha. Along with soy and corn, he also grows alfalfa hay and raises cows and calves, and says that while he could always use more moisture, he manages, as most soy farmers do, without irrigation or, thanks to modern equipment, a large crew of farmhands. And he contributes to the United States' position as the world's leading producer of soy-beans (closely followed by Brazil).

Soybeans have been cultivated for longer than almost any crop—about five thousand years—but it wasn't until the 1700s that they were introduced to Europe (and 1804 in the United States, as a returning Yankee clipper ship's ballast, not as a food item or even a cash crop). Soybeans were then used as forage in the United States until the early 1900s, not an auspicious start for such an excellent food source. They were first used here as a popular human food source as late as the 1930s and 1940s, and now, barely two genera-tions later, soybeans are grown on more than 350,000 mostly family-owned farms, covering more than 70 million acres almost entirely in the Midwest (there are more in Iowa than in any other state). For the United States, soy is truly the bean of the last century.

Most farms grow both soy and corn simultaneously in order to spread the work and the sales over various seasons. With technological advances rapidly being made in both seeds and equipment, family farms will continue to grow ever more soy, as demand increases for the bean as a healthy, abundant protein source and the base for three of the most common processed food ingredients: shortening, lecithin, and isolated protein.

✳

Perched in a $250,000 combine, I feel like I'm sitting in the cockpit of an airliner rather than in a fully evolved tractor-planter-harvester. These wonder machines come equipped these days not only with stereos and A/C, but with GPS devices and sensors that link to computer programs that map the entire field for moisture content, crop density, and yield—by the square yard. The innards, controlled by devices with names like AccuDepth™ and Touch-Set™, are loaded with conveyors and devices for processing a variety of crops (corn, soybeans, etc.) that can be adjusted infinitely to accommodate changes in crop density and moisture, too. And all the controls are ergonomic, found in panels that line the armrests, joysticks, windshield, and dashboard in ways that Boeing could only envy. Farms that needed several tractors and half a dozen workers a generation ago now can make do with one combine and one helper, as well as an office with a powerful, up-to-date computer that not only interprets all of the combine's GPS-linked harvest data, but also spews out color-coded reports that signal problems and track productivity.

When the soy plants are a few feet high, the moisture content is low, and the pods are brown (the larger, green, tender variety you eat as edamame are not fully ripened), Anderson runs his combine over the field, sets it to strip the stems and leaves and open the pods, and fills truck after truck with soybeans, ready for shipment to the co-ops, and eventually the soybean processors.

OIL FROM GAS

Everything about oilseed processing is big. Crushing and refining plants are found throughout the Midwest, and Bunge, the world's largest oilseed processor, with 23,500 employees and annual revenues of $24 billion, operates the world's largest plant across the Missouri River in Council Bluffs, Iowa. A group of yurt-like tempering tanks, each large enough to encompass a football field, dominates the landscape. Skyscraper-size cement towers, all connected by angled, pipe-covered conveyors, are rimmed by mile-long freight trains that are dwarfed by the plant. (It takes a lot to dwarf such a freight train.) The plant processes 170,000 bushels—about four and half tons—of soybeans every day of the year. ADM, headquartered in Decatur, Illinois, handles more than 3 million bushels a day (90,000 tons daily) at its 100 plants worldwide.

Driving to ADM's headquarters, I can't help but note that the roads in this otherwise rural area feel urban, congested with non-stop lines of trucks and trains bringing in soybeans (and corn) for processing. These beans are on their way to becoming pie crusts, peanut butter, and Twinkies. Crisco® starts like this.

Ag Processing Inc.'s "crushing and refining" plant is situated near the highway that runs between the Missouri River and the nearby bluffs in St. Joseph, Missouri. Surrounded by lush farm-land dotted with well-kept farms and silos, it hardly seems out of place, and can seem unremarkable as you drive by. Merely the fourth largest American company in the refined vegetable oil field, this small kid on the block boasts nine plants that process 16,000 acres' worth of soybeans—about a million bushels—every day. And although innovative processes exist, the traditional method holds strong, as is evidenced by the approach they use here.

The manufacturing of shortening, essential of both home-baked goods and processed foods, starts with the agricultural version of a giant sauna. First, the shelled soybeans are tempered—gently heated—for a week or so in large silos located along the highway. Emerging slightly softened, they then get crushed (into precisely eight pieces if all goes well) between the two rollers of the muscular "cracking roller" machine. Next, the chunks (or chips, as some places call them) are shot into "flaking rollers," which are about six feet long and have only a paper-thin gap in between them. The rollers crush the bean chunks into round, yellowish flakes the size of cornflakes. However, instead of being uneven (or frosted), these are flat and naturally loaded with oil—oil making up about 20 percent of a soy flake. The flakes are then augured up and over to the five-story-high extraction tower, where they become shortening, lecithin, or soy protein isolate (or soy flour and the like)—but only with the help of a mildly toxic, explosive solvent, hexane, which is obtained from natural gas and is a common component of gasoline.

✳

The process is similar for soy alternatives such as cottonseed oil, sunflower oil, canola oil, and palm oil; the choice changes every few years as more discoveries concerning fat are made or laws are enacted (such as the recent mandate to label trans fats), and this is reflected in the changing Twinkies shortening ingredient list. The most recent list includes cottonseed oil, canola oil, and also the decidedly nonvegetable beef fat. (Beef fat is now a common ingredient in Twinkies, as part of the shortening blend, thanks in part to its lack of trans fats.)

The soy alternatives and partners come from all over. Numerous mills in the U.S. South press cottonseed for oil, right after a cotton gin separates the seeds from the cotton and removes the hulls from them. Canola oil is pressed from the tiny black seeds (a few millimeters in diameter) of a bright yellow flowering, leafy plant of the mustard family developed in the 1970s for its excellent nutritional profile. Most canola comes from Canada (the trade-marked name canola was coined in 1979 from the words "Canadian oil"), but close to 1.5 billion pounds a year are produced in North Dakota alone. Beef fat from slaughterhouses is dehydrated, odor-neutralized, clarified, and rendered, usually by specialized companies, into a solid white, saturated fat called tallow. And sometimes palm or palm kernel oil, from oil palm plantations in Malaysia or Indonesia, is included in the mix. These all may appear on the Twinkie label, but as parts of a blend, included to add some characteristic or to cut costs as each bean's price fluctuates. Still, soybean oil makes up 80 to 90 percent of all vegetable oils processed this way. It works admirably and it is usually the cheapest oil available, so the others are only minor players on the scene. That's why soybean oil is probably the most popular vegetable oil in home kitchens and why it is the only one described here.

✳

The hexane solvent is so flammable that the entire extraction area, an OSHA "controlled environment," is off-limits. (Even the company's own corporate types aren't allowed in.) The risk of explosion is so severe that wrenches in the plant are made of special alloys that can't cause sparks. Luckily, Maury Belcher, Director of Corporate Quality Assurance for Refined Oils, has spent years running the show and knows the off-limits parts of the Ag Inc. plant like the back of his hand. Belcher walks me through the process that most companies use, from bean to shortening.

THE FORK IS TAKEN

In the extraction tower, the oil dissolves out of the flakes and into the liquid hexane solvent, which is then boiled to evaporate (and get recycled). Hazardous solvents may seem incompatible with food, but they have a welcome habit of disappearing from it. They're volatile, after all (some critics doubt that all traces are removed, but the industry is confident that they are. The alternative is expensive, expeller-pressed oils). What's left is crude vegetable oil, a viscous, amber, beany-tasting oil along with spent flakes, now turned white due to their dried-out state. Both have a long way to go to reach usefulness.

The three Twinkies ingredients—shortening, lecithin, and soy protein isolate—emerge from one of two different paths at this point. The slightly viscous crude oil goes on to become liquid products like lecithin, salad (vegetable) oil, and shortening (in that order), while the edible, defatted flakes go through a "desolventizer toaster" that warms and softens them and ensures all the solvent is gone. The flakes go on to become soy protein concentrate, soy grits, soy flour, textured vegetable protein (veggie patties, mock chicken, etc., for Boca® and veggie burgers) or, more important, soy protein isolate for foods like tofu dogs . . . and Twinkies. As Yogi Berra might have said, the fork in the road is taken.

GLOP AND GUM

When the crude oil leaves the extraction tower, a brownish black, smelly sludge—lecithin—settles toward the bottom. These days, "lecithin" has become a generic term for a whole class of fat- and water-soluble compounds, but the guys in the biz just call it gum. And the next natural thing to do, is, well, degum it.

Happily, degumming involves something a whole lot less toxic than hexane: good old-fashioned water. Warm water is mixed into the oil, immediately absorbed by the gum, and spun out in a room full of about a dozen centrifuges, each the size of an office desk, less than an hour later. The degummed oil goes on to become vegetable oil, margarine, or, more important for Twinkies, partially hydrogenated vegetable shortening. What's left is a dark brown thick glop—that's actually the technical term—from which the added water is slowly removed through gentle heating.

When the glop resembles molasses, it is ready for bakeries or other food companies to process further for their clients (some make "refined" lecithin by bleaching it and/or removing the remaining oil with acetone, the same solvent found in nail polish remover). Others clarify it for use in the nutritional supplement capsules you can buy at the health food store.

Lecithin, discovered in 1805, when French scientist Maurice Gobley identified it in egg yolks, is found in trace amounts in almost all living cells. Lecithin makes up an astonishing 30 percent of the yolk in an egg, as opposed to 1.5 to 3 percent in soybeans. That must be why Monsieur Gobley named it after the Greek word for "egg yolk," *lekithos*.

It is not easy to extract lecithin from egg yolks, but for years no one knew where else it could be found. And it was likely worth a search, considering the amazing capacity for egg yolks to emulsify, best demonstrated by the ability of one yolk to absorb more than a cup of oil to make mayonnaise. Cooking guru Shirley O. Corriher calls egg yolk the "superemulsifier." Whip up some mayo in your kitchen, if you haven't done so before, and you'll no doubt be impressed.

Soybean oil processing became popular in Europe after 1908, during which refiners found themselves with a stinky, residual waste sludge. In 1920, German food scientists, examining that waste for hidden assets, identified it as lecithin. ADM started refining it in Chicago, under German license, in 1934. By 1939, the Germans had come up with more than a thousand new uses for it. Considering that it's separated with only water and force, and that it is still "all-natural," it's a darn good deal.

Lecithin's primary job in Twinkies, as well as in most foods, is to emulsify, or tie water and fat together, on a molecular level. Each molecule has two tails, one of which targets fat, the other of which gloms on to water. Because of this unique ability, and because it has been around for so long, it's practically ubiquitous in processed foods. Lecithin is also famous for being one of the first emulsifiers to be used in baked goods, starting in the 1920s. One of the most widely used, naturally occurring emulsifiers in the world, lecithin is often paired (as it is in Twinkies) with its synthetic counterparts, mono and diglycerides and the more modern polysorbate 60, in order to emulsify a wider range of water and oil mixtures.

In addition, lecithin does a lot more than simply blend fat and water. In the annals of Great Accomplishments, lecithin serves a purpose for which I'd bet many of us are especially grateful: it makes chocolate smooth and prevents "bloom" (fat) on the surface. Look at almost any chocolate bar label, even the very best, and there it is. As if that weren't enough to make it our favorite ingredient on the Twinkie label, it also binds and smooths out ingredients in ice cream, chewing gum, and peanut butter. It even helps keep margarine from spattering when heated. Lecithin makes batters easier to mix and cuts down on lumping. It whips toppings, whitens coffee, smooths out processed cheese, fills out ice cream cones and waffle mixes, and even helps disperse dry beverage mixes. In bread, it's essential to just about everything: distribution of shortening, dough handling, moisture retention, texture, volume, and shelf life ("anti-staling"—it reduces crumb firming). But its greatest contribution is when it functions as an egg yolk replacement and "egg yolk sparing agent" (as it's known). Certainly, that is its most distinctive function in Twinkies—another way to cut down on ingredients that might spoil. Also, like egg yolks, it invites the gentle, uniform browning of Twinkies' bottom (the top, in reality), and keeps the texture of the crumb soft yet strong enough to stay together.

The fact that it comes from a vegetarian source is an added bonus, and why it's listed on the Twinkie ingredient label as "soy lecithin"—to distinguish it from "chicken" lecithin extracted from eggs. Lecithin can be included on the label of an "all-natural" food product, which accounts for a lot of its popularity, and almost all the major producers make it certified kosher. Though it functions primarily as an emulsifier, it is also called a wetting agent, an "instantizer" (helping things dissolve), a release agent (in PAM® cooking spray), a viscosity modifier, a mixing aid, an antidusting agent, and more. It is high in polyunsaturates and is cholesterol-free and totally safe to eat.

Lecithin is big in industry, too. It's an excellent pigment dispersant in paints, water-based printing inks, plastic, and even videotapes (it's known as a surfactant, not an emulsifier, in the paint and coating industry). It softens the skin when blended into cosmetics, helps oil penetrate leather, and plays a role in paper coating, waxes, caulks, adhesives, lubricants, and explosives. All in all, a rather impressive, wonderful range of uses for a former waste product.

These days, scientists are looking for ways to make new lecithin products by modifying it genetically and enzymatically, and by using filtration, compounding, and other specialized techniques. But it seems satisfying enough (for our purposes, at least) that it is used in Twinkies.

As good as lecithin is, it pales by comparison in usefulness to the most important soy product of all, partially hydrogenated vegetable shortening, the next item made in this production line.

The French Connection

It's a long way to shortening, and a long way from France.
The newly degummed oil leaving the lecithin station is still

crude. Before it can become shortening, even now that it is light-
ened of its lecithin, it must be leavened, meaning refined, bleached,
and deodorized.

We consumers like our oils clear, so the crude oil, after being
cleansed with a hit of sodium hydroxide (caustic soda), is mixed
with a claylike product that removes chlorophyll and the remaining carotenoid pigments that color it yellow. We also like our oils
tasteless and deodorized, so next the oil is heated to about 500°F
for up to an hour under virtually a vacuum—vaporizing any remaining free fatty acids, off-flavors, and moisture. Blasts of steam
remove any residual leftovers. Finally, the oil achieves the light,
bland color and consistency that we like to use at home—for salad
dressings, baking, and frying. Beyond food, some will end up in
an amazing array of industrial goods, including (after more processing, of course) alkyd paints—the current version of oil paint—
rubber, caulk, adhesive tape, leather softeners, and, surprisingly,
diesel fuel. And all of it stems from a simple bean.

It takes about six hours to turn beans into salad oil, which is an
ambitious feat. But it's at this point in the process where oil refining
gets really interesting. Plain vegetable oil, despite being 100 percent
fat, is a pourable liquid. What the bakeries seek is a soft solid that
resembles butter or lard. The magic happens in turning a liquid
into a solid, which apparently isn't as hard as it sounds, so long as
you have the knowledge and the equipment to force some hydrogen molecules into it. Hydrogenation creates a semisolid oil that
behaves like butter[8] but costs a whole lot less, contains as much as
50 percent less saturated fat, and is so stable that it doesn't require
refrigeration for up to a year. That's a shelf life. And that's Crisco®.

An oil to which only *some* hydrogen has been added is called

---

8. Most important, shortening has a much higher melting point than butter,
more akin to lard's, so it acts as a space holder to create air pockets in cakes or pie
shells, making them tender and flaky.

partially hydrogenated. Oils that are even more lightly hydro-genated are liquid shortenings; an oil with as much hydrogen as chemically possible added is called "fully hydrogenated" and is as solid as candle wax (you can actually buy candles made of veg-etable oil, called stearin, or "soy" candles, which burn more cleanly than traditional candle wax, which is mostly made of paraffin, a petroleum product). All it takes is high heat, high pressure, a maze of steel towers, and a dose of hydrogen.

In a hydrogenation facility, upward of 60,000 pounds of the newly refined oil is pumped into a pipe-covered, two- to three-story-high, pressurized, vertical tank called a converter, where it is heated to over 400°F while hydrogen gas is pumped in under 150 pounds per square inch (psi) pressure, along with a catalyst in the form of a bunch of little metal (nickel) balls that look like BBs. The whole operation is so hot that it has to be located outside the plant building, and I can only observe from a safe distance. The mixture is stirred by several large propellers on a central shaft, which means the converters are really nothing more than giant blenders. The oil becomes hydrogenated in this way, but it's not quite shortening yet.

Depending on how solid the desired outcome, and depend-ing on the beans themselves (affected as they are by the growing season's rainfall, sun, and average temperatures), the chefs (aka engineers) in the control room cook the mixture for anywhere from fifteen minutes to two hours. They can make it pourable, brushable, spreadable, or hard as soap—each batch is made to or-der in this giant, industrial café.

Shortening as we know it is not made in one tank in one batch—that would be too simple—but is a blend of partially and sometimes fully hydrogenated oils and up to 80 percent unhy-drogenated, liquid oil. The solid, edible, hydrogenated oil forms a honeycomb framework into which the liquid oil seeps, just like a honeycomb holds honey. As it happens, hydrogenated soybean and canola oils boast the most stable and dense crystalline structure (hence the highest melting and smoke point) of all of the fats, while palm oil's looser structure makes it easier to incorporate air during mixing. That is one reason all three oils show up on the Twinkies ingredient list (the other reason is pricing and availability).

The same process is used for hydrogenating two other Twinkies subingredients: stearic acid (which is used in polysorbate 60 and sodium stearoyl lactylate) and sorbitol (which is used in polysorbate 60).

When the proportions are right, the shortening is blended with emulsifiers (mono and diglycerides, which are also used on their own in Twinkies) to make it water-friendly and to raise the melting point—two characteristics required for baking. (Add lots of water, some artificial flavors and colors, more emulsifiers, and preservatives, and you've got margarine; add even more water and you've got Dairy Fresh Non-Dairy Creamer.™) The shortening then gets whipped while being chilled to introduce as much air (and sometimes nitrogen) as possible, air that will later be trapped in batter to make an airy Twinkie, pie crust, or creamy filling.

Wouldn't you know it? We have the French to thank for this magnificent culinary achievement, which enables us to enjoy fine, packaged pastries for a dollar a hit. Hydrogenation was invented in 1905 by French chemist Paul Sabatier. (Procter & Gamble claims the title, though, saying they developed it in 1907 with a German scientist.) In 1912, Sabatier won the Nobel Prize in Chemistry for discovering that nickel (along with platinum) is a good hydrogenation catalyst. Crisco—then made from cottonseed oil (its name, selected in a Procter & Gamble employee contest, is a near-acronym derived from *cry*stalized *c*ottonseed *oil*)—came on the market in 1911, pitched even then by Procter & Gamble as a healthy alternative to butter and lard. In 1913, it sent a team of home economists around the country to demonstrate cooking with Crisco, with much success. Well into the twenty-first century, shortening made of partially hydrogenated oils was still seen as a godsend, until research began to reveal that it was almost killing us.

What You Don't Know Can Kill You

While the actual hydrogenation process is relatively simple, the science and technology behind it is not.

All fat molecules are made of long chains of carbon atoms (among other things). In oils (fats that are liquid at room temperature) most carbon atoms have two hydrogen atoms attached to their two "arms." Those carbon atoms that have only one hydrogen atom attached have, therefore, an available arm for another hydrogen atom to attach itself. When hydrogen atoms are forced onto only some of the available carbon atoms' arms, the oil becomes a little more solid, or "partially hydrogenated." If hydrogen atoms are forced onto every one of the available carbon atoms' arms, the oil becomes solid and is called "fully hydrogenated."

What's important to know from a health perspective is that the molecules in unsaturated fats—most vegetable fats, such as those in salad oils—are shaped in a way that is supposedly easily digested by our bodies. On the other hand, the molecules found in saturated fats—naturally occurring in animal fats such as butter, tallow (beef fat), and lard (pork fat) that shortening is supposed to replace—are shaped in a way that many authorities think is not easily digested by the body and therefore, some believe, raise our "bad" cholesterol by converting into artery-clogging plaque.

Alarmingly, unpredictable events have been known to transpire during the hydrogenation process—things neither the scientists nor the engineers can control nor fully explain. Hydrogen atoms have been known to "jump" across the molecule creating what we call trans fats ("trans" means "across"; "trans fats" is short for "trans-fatty acids"), resulting in slightly deformed molecules. When this happens, you're left with an oil that behaves like a solid, a fat that not only raises bad cholesterol but lowers the good. Since January 1, 2006, federal law has mandated that trans fats be noted on the Nutrition Facts label of all packaged foods, which has caused many a manufacturer to change their recipes—Twinkies included.

When hydrogenating oils, reducing or eliminating trans fats is a challenge, causing the guys in the control room and the folks at the labs to work hard to manipulate the temperature, pressure, ingredients, and timing that, even in the best possible circumstances, does affect the shortening's texture, melting point, and cost. Crisco seems to have pulled it off by including high-oleic sunflower oil and continuing the hydrogenation process about twenty or thirty minutes longer until the soybean oil is fully hydrogenated, or fully saturated (meaning there is no space for trans fats on the molecules), then mixing a little bit of it with unhydrogenated oil. Iowa State University has spent thirty years developing an ultralow linolenic soybean that requires no hydrogenation; some European food companies have changed their shortening recipe by mixing in palm oil or beef fat, which are naturally highly saturated, obviating the need for partial hydrogenation and avoiding the creation of trans fats.[9] Young food scientists (along with their employers) dream of finding the "killer app" of ingredients, the perfectly healthy, guilt-free, fat substitute.

---

9. This explains why beef fat showed up on more Twinkies ingredient labels in 2006 (it appeared less often before), and why the shortening is now called "vegetable and/or animal shortening." That's why Twinkies are no longer kosher, not that all of them were. Apparently only one or two of the various Hostess bakeries made kosher Twinkies, for what it's worth. Kosher foods are often viewed by consumers who don't need to eat kosher foods as slightly better than nonkosher foods, even snack cakes, somewhat akin to the way "all natural" labels boost sales on things like ice cream.

We will always, it seems, strive for the best of all possible worlds in our quest for the perfect cake.

Creamy Oil

In the thick of such complex science, it's important to step back and appreciate that the goal, at the end of the day, is simply to make a better form of fat. You need fat in cake to make it tender, light, and delicate, and, as in all foods, to carry flavors and nutrients. Butter may have better flavor, but it doesn't leaven as well as our favorite heavily processed soybean product.

The primary advantage of shortening is that its high melting point and crystalline structure ensure an airy cake or a flaky crust. But shortening offers another advantage: it makes cakes tender by coating the flour proteins with oil, keeping them from absorbing moisture, and "shortening" (hence the term) the gluten strands. Try tearing a piece off a crusty boule of peasant bread, which has plenty of gluten, and compare that heroic effort with the effort needed to tear off a piece of cake. Twinkies are so tender, the hardest thing to tear off is the wrapper.

Shortening's also essential to providing some slippery fat in the Twinkie filling, where it is whipped up with water, sugar, corn syrup, and a host of emulsifiers and thickeners. (That famous creamy filling has no cream in it, of course, which is why it is spelled "creme.") Partially hydrogenated vegetable shortening is one of the main ingredients in cremelike products, such as Kraft's Cool Whip® non-dairy whipped topping and ready-made cake icings. It's found in some brands of peanut butter (or fully hydrogenated oil, in order to avoid trans fats).

Fat not only shortens the dough in Twinkies, it holds the batter together. It tenderizes, moisturizes, and aerates the crumb, and gives both the cake and the filling a nice, rich mouthfeel. What more could you want in a snack?

ISOLATION

Soybeans are considered healthful because they are such an excellent source of protein. So it would seem that isolating that protein would be useful in a variety of food products. As if processing the oil into shortening and lecithin weren't enough, at least one company has staked its future on specialized products such as soy protein isolate: the Solae Company, in St. Louis, Missouri, created by food and technology giants Bunge and DuPont.

A crusher plant like Ag Processing ships its oil-less flakes across the state to Solae, where the softened flakes are dumped, a liquid railcar's worth at a time (more than 20,000 gallons), into a vat of warm water and lye (or lime, ammonia, or tribasic phosphate), creating a soggy mess akin to a thin milk shake. After about an hour of gentle agitation, the proteins and sugars are dissolved and the protein can be extracted in an airplane hangarlike building full of centrifuges, ranging in size from that of a small up to a full-size car.

The second step is a lot like making cheese. A bit of acid, usually hydrochloric, is added to the moist mix in a 4,000- or 5,000-gallon tank, which triggers a curdling reaction, somewhat like how tofu is made. In an ironic twist for this well-known dairy alternative, the proteins are called curds and the watery effluent whey.

Finally, the third step is to dry the soy protein into the desired shapes and sizes—finely powdered for drinks and baking, larger for soy "meat." Three tons of flakes make one ton of isolated protein, explaining why it costs about five to seven times as much as soy flour. What makes it so valuable is that it's 90 to 95 percent protein—a superior concentration to soy flour that makes it useful in a lot more items than cake. Soy protein isolate finds its way into frankfurters and bologna, to help bind fat and moisture for added firmness and also to replace more expensive meat and dairy proteins. It is a central player in soy-based infant formulas and dietetic or nutritional meal supplements. It boosts the protein content of many commercial bread brands as well as pasta, and provides a nondairy, cholesterol-free, all-vegetarian alternative additive for coffee whiteners, whipped toppings, Power Bars®, and bacon bits. In Japan, it is part of surimi, the "restructured fish product" that we know as fake crabmeat or "sea legs," most often found in California rolls. One of its greatest attributes is that it has no taste, so it's infinitely adaptable. And, like so many of the other Twinkie ingredients, soy protein isolate has industrial applications as well, including binding the shiny clay coatings on cereal boxes.

Given its myriad manifestations, it would appear that you can't bake Twinkies without soybeans, a plant that barely registered on Western consciousness a hundred years ago. Soybeans in cake. Who knew?

But certainly you'd expect a cake to contain eggs.

CHAPTER 11

-- -- -- -- -- -- --

Eggs

Twinkies bakeries use a million eggs a year. Imagine if the bakers actually had to break each and every one of them by hand! In this mighty industrialized process, the big bakeries simply buy eggs that are already broken—dried, liquid, or frozen—from companies that do nothing but break eggs. Turns out that egg-breaking is big business.

I had never, ever even remotely imagined that there exists in this world a specialized industry for egg-breaking, so nothing prepared me for Papetti's Hygrade Egg Products, the country's largest egg-breaking facility, in Elizabeth, New Jersey.

Papetti's breaks 7 million eggs a day at its New Jersey plant, located in an industrial park near Newark Airport. The mere idea of breaking, let alone handling, that many eggs, even over a lifetime, is hard for a mere mortal to conceive. But here at Papetti's, big tractor-trailers arrive hourly and tank trucks depart almost as often, each loaded with 6,000 gallons of fresh, whole, liquid eggs. It is the largest egg plant in the country, and we're not talking a prize-winner at a state fair. Its corporate parent, Michael Foods, processes more eggs than anyone else in the world.

Miracle Glue

Whole eggs are the last item listed on the Twinkie label before the "2% or less" category, so, much to my surprise (not really), there isn't a lot of egg in a Twinkie. A "scratch" sponge cake recipe calls for a quarter of an egg or more per Twinkie-size cake. (A little math based on the figures cited on Hostess's Web site claims they use 1 million eggs to make the 500 million Twinkies they sell each year, which equals 1/500th of an egg per Twinkie, or two-tenths of 1 percent. But eggs are more prominent on the ingredient list than that figure indicates, and Hostess won't confirm either way.) Nutrition isn't the point of including eggs in cakes like Twinkies—they're there because they are the glue that holds everything together.

Eggs leaven cake in a variety of ways, helping to structure the dough by serving as a binder or emulsifier, holding oil and water together in the form of a nice crumb. The yolk's fat (about five grams in a large egg) acts like a lubricant, softening the dough's texture. Egg white is almost entirely pure protein, and, especially once it is whipped, helps leaven the batter by creating and maintaining bubbles when it is baked. (Twinkies, of course, use chemical leavening, unlike a true sponge cake.) Toward the end of a cake's baking time, the fat and protein in the egg yolk and white contribute to browning through the Maillard reactions, where sugar and the egg's amino acids, notably lysine, react with heat and turn the cake brown in a series of complex chemical reactions.

However, as we know, Twinkies are meant to have a long shelf life, and eggs normally present problems of spoilage from mold. The bakeries meet this challenge by using mostly dried eggs, which lessens both the moisture level and the microbe risk. And, of course, the food scientists at Hostess have thrown a whole bagful of tricks at this problem in their Olympian efforts to extend shelf life, using a combination of lots of sugar, a dash of salt, and a smidgeon of a powerful preservative called sorbic acid. The eggs found in Twinkies are as good as dead, as far as microbes are concerned.

The egg business is evidently a good one. Papetti's makes more than three hundred egg products, some of which are remixed in different percentages of yolk or white for clients' recipes or budgets, or as a low-cholesterol product. The combined egg mixture—or just yolks or just whites—is packaged in cardboard cartons after processing in order to extend its grocery store shelf life up to an astounding twelve weeks, versus six weeks for shell eggs, and that's pushing it.

Papetti's goes way beyond plain egg products. The rest of the egg mixture in the New Jersey plant is preprocessed for various food companies by mixing in ingredients like sugar, corn syrup (for ice cream), salt, and nonfat dried milk. The fresh, frozen, and processed egg customers include some of the best-known national brands of ice cream (such as Ben & Jerry's, which buys yolks for flavor enhancement and rich taste), pasta (Ronzoni®—yolks, mostly for color but also richer taste), cakes (Entenmann's—whites for leavening and crumb, yolks for taste and browning), mayonnaise (Hellmann's—yolks, as an emulsifier), and cookies (Famous Amos®—whole eggs for flavor and browning), dozens of whose packages are proudly displayed in Papetti's lobby.

Eggs (in some cases just the whites, in others, just the yolks) also bind meat and fish in loaves or croquettes, thicken custards and sauces, emulsify mayonnaise-based sauces and dressings, coat or glaze breads, clarify soups and coffee, retard crystallization in candies and frosting, and leaven soufflés and, of course, sponge cakes (added emulsifiers do these jobs in Twinkies). Egg promoters call eggs "the cement that holds the castle of cuisine together." With reason.

Breaking Point

Egg-breaking starts with a riot of colors in the loading area. John Gill, Papetti's plant manager, offers a warm welcome and escorts me into a chilly (45°F) reception area the size of an airplane hangar, where pallets of egg cases, as they call the plastic trays, are being unloaded from trucks and stacked. The cases, which are made from randomly colored recycled plastic, are green, red, yellow, and black today, in stark contrast to the white of the eggs that peek through. Each case holds thirty eggs. There are thousands of them here, with a thousand arriving or being removed at every moment (no eggs stay here for more than a few hours).

About twenty-five tractor-trailers arrive throughout the day, each filled with more than 22,500 dozen eggs, fresh from regional farms. As you might imagine, the forklift operators must have a delicate touch and a goodly amount of self-assurance, as they move stacks of well over a thousand eggs at once with nary a nick.

The stacks meld the natural with the industrial: next to the bar codes that track the eggs' industrial origin in minute detail, the occasional feather and bit of straw reveal their rural origin. These are fresh; some, hatched barely a day ago, are called nesters. Of course, in order to have eggs, you gotta have chickens.

Which Came First?

The chicken. That takes care of *that*.

Egg farms that supply the Elizabeth facility are scattered throughout Pennsylvania, western New Jersey, and Ohio. Some are small, with as few as 50,000 hens in one long, low henhouse, while others top out at more than 300,000 layers. The average egg farm contains about 100,000 hens. Most are small, family farmers working under contract to supply unbroken eggs to the big egg-processing company. (The larger, corporate facilities in the Midwest break eggs right at the farm for drying and freezing.)

The hens are all Leghorns, bred for their remarkable egg-laying ability (unlike their country cousins, the big-breasted hens that are bred for food). No visitors are allowed in the henhouse, for fear of infection that could spread quickly among so many chickens in such close quarters. And while the exclusion of visitors is first and foremost for the chickens' safety, it strikes me as a good idea. The inside of a crowded henhouse is simply not somewhere you want to be.

The hens arrive as day-old chicks or fourteen- to eighteen-week-old pullets (teenagers) and start laying eggs after about eighteen weeks. They require twenty-one to twenty-six hours to lay an egg, and they dutifully produce good, solid eggs daily, if all goes well, until they are about seventy weeks old (about sixteen months). Some farmers take them out of the egg-laying rotation for about a month at this point in order to let their systems rebuild calcium supplies (via reduced light and a change in feed). After that they might lay for another eight months or so, until they're about two years old. "Spent hens," as they're called, are not good candidates for packaged chicken meat intended for supermarket shelves because they're pretty scrawny, weighing about half of a "meat" chicken. So after contributing their best eggs to the Twinkies cause, the hens end up in chicken soup, nuggets, patties, pet food, and pig feed.

The hens spend their days in a controlled environment, eating a powdered feed that is usually about two-thirds corn and a quarter soybean meal, plus calcium, salt, and various micronutrients that include amino acids (such as lysine), vitamins, and minerals. Some farms grow corn and soybeans nearby expressly for chicken feed, supplying the mixture by a conveyor connecting the two facilities. The lights are carefully manipulated to maximize egg-laying with an optimum day-night cycle, and the cages are tilted seven degrees so that the freshly laid eggs roll right onto a conveyor belt that runs continuously (and gently) alongside the cages.

Most hens lay their eggs by morning, but some dillydally about until noon. These eggs are moved via conveyor to merge with a flow of eggs from a larger conveyor that brings all of them to a packing head where workers place them onto the colorful trays that are eventually delivered ever so carefully to Elizabeth. Surprisingly, the eggs usually survive their trip quite well. It's the loading and unloading where things can easily get messy.

IF YOU WANT AN OMELET . . .

Around the corner from the chilly unloading area, the machines take over. They are not without human company, but people are clearly the minority.

First, the eggs are conveyed in stacks, from which steel arms pluck individual trays and align them for washing and sanitizing. The machine that accomplishes this at this facility is quite similar to the kind of dishwasher you would find in any large restaurant kitchen, only it's over sixty-five feet long. Then, the eggs are picked up thirty at a time by mechanical arms (dotted with suction cups) and placed precisely in rows of dozens on a wide, slow conveyor that is part of another continuous, giant washing machine. A bright light underneath allows for inspection through the shells by sharp-eyed monitors.

These busy human teammates are mostly women who carefully pluck out bad eggs (cracked or fertilized) and deftly replace them with good ones so that the conveyor stays full as it moves along. The bad eggs, called inedibles (as in "not suitable for human consumption"), get dropped quickly into a familiar-looking, low-tech device called a "bucket" designated for the sideline production of pet food. A small silo out back is reserved solely for these outcasts.

One by one, the rows of eggs fall off the end of the conveyor like Rockettes taking a bow. Each egg falls into a cup on a giant spinning wheel that's part of the aptly named "egg breaking-and-separating machine," which is whirring at blur speed despite its ten-foot diameter and eight-foot height. There are two rows of cups on some half a dozen machines of various sizes and customized designs. On one machine, the egg is immediately seized on each oval end by two small suction cups. The supporting cup falls away, and the fun begins.

Picture one egg among many suspended on a whizzing carousel, and follow the process as you walk around the wheel: a knife shoots up to give the egg a surgical whack, slicing cleanly through the shell. It then falls back into position, ready for the next hit a second later. Suction cups pull the shell halves back and up at a slight angle, perfectly mimicking the gesture countless cooks make in their kitchens as they crack eggs one by one. The yolk and white drop down into a set of corresponding cups. As the yolk plops down into a small, appropriately sized upper cup, the white falls down around it into a funnel cup, just underneath. Gentle blasts of air coax the last of the egg out of its shell, and the yolk cups are bounced a bit to shake the white completely out—again, much like you do at home.

As the giant wheel spins, both yolk and white pass through electronic scanners that zero in on shell bits, white in the yolk, or yolk in the white. Some very focused attendants supervise them. As the wheel whirls toward the end of its revolution, the cups tip into two open stainless steel troughs (if separate egg parts are desired), or one (if the goal is whole eggs). The shells are spun off into oblivion, destined to be dried and ground into fertilizer for local farmers, and the suction cups position themselves for the next round of eggs a split second later. The whole process takes less than ten seconds.

Different breaker-separator machines work at different speeds, and some are reputed to break well over 140,000 eggs per hour. When I'm showing my daughter how to break eggs with essentially the same motions, it takes us about a minute just to break one.

Pumping and pasteurizing eggs through the jungle of narrow, highly polished stainless steel pipes take no less a delicate touch than it takes to handle shell eggs, as failure to maintain the right combination of time, temperature, and movement in those pipes could spell disaster in the form of a three-inch-diameter omelet dozens of yards long. After a flash pasteurization process and a quick homogenization, the egg mixture is pumped through an array of chilled, sterile silos ranging in size from 5,000 to 20,000 gallons. From there, liquid eggs are pumped into sterilized tank trucks, which are insulated but not cooled (this would only pose a problem if the truck got stalled for a few days in a huge traffic jam on a hot day in August with close to 50,000 pounds of raw eggs inside). Some customers take them in 2,000-pound plastic boxes sized to fit on pallets; others prefer "just-in-time" delivery, which involves pumping the eggs directly from the tanker into a mixing vat. Now that's fresh. Sort of. The nesters are history less than an hour after leaving the truck.

Not all of the freshly broken eggs are shipped out in raw form (the preferred form among the higher-end products): some of the mixture is frozen (often a second choice in flavor quality), and, at other facilities, much of it is dried. The broken eggs sent to the freezing plant are mixed with corn syrup or salt (eggs will not freeze well without one of these) and then frozen in thirty-pound, five-gallon buckets for big bakers such as Twinkies and Sara Lee. In the Elizabeth plant, some of the liquid egg mixture is channeled directly into a nearby kitchen, where it is cooked into uniform oval, half-inch-thick omelets and frozen for use by school cafeterias and major fast-food chains. If you want a few million omelets, you've got to break a few million eggs.

Nebraska Dried

The Elizabeth facility thrives on variety, but Michael Foods' Wakefield, Nebraska, plant is the principal source for dried eggs. This is one of the biggest laying facilities in the world, with about 4 million hens laying eggs daily, all under the watchful eye of Tim Bebee, Vice President of Live Production. What with the plant located in the Midwest, shipment to either coast is long and obviously not advised for unbroken "shell" eggs. So the eggs are broken on-site at the chicken houses, using the same process as in the Elizabeth, New Jersey, plant, and dried just a short tank truck ride away. There, tiny droplets of pasteurized egg are sprayed into the tops of multiple hot-air box dryers twenty feet tall, thirty feet deep, and fifty feet long. Before your very eyes, dried eggs fall to the bottom as a powder, and are promptly packed into fifty-pound boxes or bags for shipping to bakeries or cafeterias.

A big bakery such as one that makes Twinkies might require dried or frozen eggs as well as liquid eggs, separated or in various yolk/white blends depending on recipe changes, pricing, or the equipment on hand. Each form of egg product requires its own recipe or handling adjustment: fresh eggs need refrigeration; frozen eggs need freezers and time to thaw; and the chef must know to compensate for the added salt or sugar.

Dried eggs, with their lack of moisture and subsequent resistance to spoilage, are actually more practical for use in a product with a long shelf life, like the Twinkie. Being relatively shelf stable, dried eggs are by far the easiest, cheapest, and safest form to handle (no refrigeration or freezing needed, thus almost no worry of contamination). That's why it is likely that the vast majority of eggs used in cakes these days are dried, primarily due to safety issues, but also due to the obvious cost-effectiveness. They are easier to use than other forms, too. The powder is simply mixed into the dough at the outset—there's no need for separate rehydration; merely add a little extra water to the batter and a little extra time to soak it up.

Though scrambled eggs made from powder never taste quite like fresh eggs, dried eggs work quite well in a baked item in which they are a minor ingredient and all of the other ingredients work together to disguise any "off" flavors. All of the other functions that eggs perform remain apparently intact.

Industry professionals may promote their product as the "incredible, edible egg," but what's incredible, in fact, is egg harvesting, from the seven-degree slant of a nester's cage to the whirling carousel that mimics a chef's gesture. And, of course, there are those trucks full of eggs, six thousand gallons of raw eggs careening down the highway. Given that nearly everyone's made a cake with eggs, it's not hard to imagine eggs in Twinkies. It's a lot harder to picture cotton—or trees—as cake ingredients. But that they are.

CHAPTER 12

Cellulose Gum

Cellulose is literally everywhere. It is, in fact, one of the most abundant, renewable, natural resources in the world, or, more accurately, in our biosphere. All green plants synthesize it to make their cell walls, making their stems and leaf veins rigid and fork-resistant—good sources of fiber in your diet. And though cellulose is stiff when chemically cooked, highly purified, and transformed into cellulose gum, it makes an incredibly soft goop that is perfect for lending viscosity to the filling in snack cakes—or rocket fuel.

Cellulose gum is one of the few ingredients on the Twinkies label with no real "home equivalent." In fact, the closest you'd come to mimicking the job of cellulose gum at home is wrapping your pudding, sauce, or cake tightly and putting it in the fridge, or tossing some gelatin into your whipped cream to keep it from slumping. Hard to believe it comes from cotton and trees.

Even though cellulose gum is more of a modern food additive, our interest in plain, basic cellulose as a chemical began more than a century ago.

FROM FILM TO PHARMACEUTICALS

Germany in the late 1800s was a hotbed of scientific creativity, and the search for a suitable material for photographic film by the old Kodak competitor, Agfa (the company that invented color film), may have led to the discovery of just how to extract cellulose acetate from a wood pulp soup. German chemical giant IG Farben then took it a bit further. Looking to make artificial silk, Farben synthesized cellulose gum in its labs to end up with rayon, first produced on a major scale in Germany in 1934 (a patent was issued in 1918). Meanwhile, in the United States, Dow Chemical had begun making cellophane from cellulose in 1927, which was followed by ethyl cellulose, its first plastic resin, in 1935 (better known for its use in items like luggage, hard hats, hairbrushes, and flashlight cases, ethyl cellulose is fortunately not found in Twinkies). However indirectly, the invention of rayon and ethyl cellulose led to the use of cellulose in food, until World War II put a stop to the German export of cellulose to the United States.

In the 1960s, with the drive for less expensive and lower-fat processed foods, cellulose gum found its way into foods like ice cream, as well as pharmaceutical and personal care products like toothpaste. Today, cellulose gum's popularity continues to grow multifold. And there is no problem finding a good supply of the raw material. You don't have to pump it out of the ground in the Middle East.

You can just grow it.

COOKING BLOTTER PAPER

Both trees and cotton are farmed sources of cellulose gum, but each has its own strengths and limitations. Tree farming, for example, may be the slowest farming in the world. It takes about twenty or twenty-five years for a crop of "fast-growing" pine or spruce trees to reach market size—about nine inches in diameter at breast height. After a year or so, seedlings don't require much in the way of weeding or herbicides. Fertilizing is suggested only once or twice a generation, something most lawn owners would love.

Private landowners grow most of the pine in the Southeast (in fact, most U.S. forestland is privately owned), and most of those tree farms—typically less than five hundred acres—can be found in southeast Georgia and northeast Florida; you can see rows and rows of farmed pines from Route 95 just below the Georgia-Florida border. A lot of families, especially those who can trace their plantation ownership back generations, have switched from cotton or peanuts to trees, thanks in part to federal subsidies and the extraordinarily attractive advantage of having to harvest the crop only every (human) generation or so, rather than every year. Good timber management encourages traditional wildlife (and hunting) in the area, and there is a constant market for pulpwood. It's a nice life, albeit a little on the quiet side. One fifth-generation landowner and tree farmer, Don Bell, of Albany, Georgia, says, "I just enjoy seeing the trees grow."

In big wood-growing regions (the U.S. Southeast has been called "the wood basket of the world"), softwood trees from the region are stripped of their bark and branches and turned into what appear to be telephone poles—for about an instant. A noisy fury of a machine reduces them in no time to quarter-inch-thick chips about one or two inches square. At the so-called dissolving pulp mills (only about three are left in the United States), such as Rayonier in Jessup, Georgia, and Fernandina Beach, Florida, or Tembec in Temiscaming, Quebec, the chips undergo a chemical pulping process in house-size vats called digesters (just as wood is pulped for paper, pressure cooked in a treatment with acids and bleaches), which dissolve the lignin (the glue that holds the fibers together) so that it and the other chemical component of wood, hemicellulose, can be extracted. The difference between pulping for food and pulping for paper is the purity—food-grade pulp must be made to exacting specifications and, one hopes, without traces of harmful chemicals.

Unlike trees, most domestic cotton is grown on large family farms that average around three thousand acres. Also, cotton goes through a few more (and more expensive) levels of processing before it is turned into pulp. No longer a labor-intensive business, thanks to modern equipment, cotton farming is now capital-intensive: a John Deere mechanical picker can cost well over $300,000. These machines look a bit like combines, equipped with special fingers several feet long that protrude from the front of the machine in order to gather the crop from the plants as they move over the field.

Farmers like Allen Helms, of Marion, Arkansas, need only four or five helpers at harvesttime to run the machines. Helms has grown cotton on this land near the Mississippi River, opposite Memphis, for thirty-six years. His season is a bit shorter and more labor-intensive than the tree "season"—he plants every year in late April or early May and harvests from late September through October, as is typical across the deep South. The plant's twiggy stems, which can grow as long as eighteen inches, are not harvested, but simply ground up and dug back into the soil. Helms's trusty mechanical picker spits out giant loaves of cotton, bales (with the decidedly unfolksy name of "modules") the size of trucks, thirty-two feet long, eight feet high, and eight feet wide, which are hauled off, one at a time, to the local cotton gin.

Hundreds of gins—small factories, really—are scattered across the South, especially in Mississippi, Texas, and Arkansas. These gins separate the cotton fibers from the seeds, so that the long cotton fibers can be transported to cotton textile spinning mills to become blue jeans, while the fuzzy, peanut-size seeds travel by the truckload, perhaps several hundred miles, to a cottonseed oil mill, such as the Planters Cotton Oil Mill in Pine Bluff, down in south central Arkansas.

Before Planters crushes them for their valuable oil, machines full of spinning blades defuzz the seeds. That fuzz, the linters or "seed hair," is almost 100 percent cellulose, and, however unpalatable that may sound, the target for Twinkies. After cutting and cleaning, these fibers remain light brown, yellow, red, or even green, and Planters Cotton Oil Mill ships six-hundred-pound, three-foot-long bales of them—each less than two millimeters long—by the trainload from Pine Bluff to processors like Buckeye Technologies in Memphis, or ADM in Chattanooga, Tennessee. There, the linters get digested the same way wood chips do.

Once the fibers have come this far, whether from wood or from cotton, they are processed somewhat the same way, though cotton fibers are cooked once more in enormous digester vats, until the desired fiber length and molecular weight—breakdown—is achieved. Next: bleaching (in a warm, caustic soda solution) and washing (to remove the soda). Some plants do this at a rate of forty tons an hour, day in and day out, all in the name of creating inexpensive food.

The resulting mush is dried on wide screens, which are actually created for paper-making. Formed into sheets of what appear to be thick blotter paper, they are then cut into four-foot-square sheets or rolled onto one- to three-foot-wide spools about nine feet in diameter that weigh as much as 1,200 pounds (pros often refer to them, charmingly, as "giant rolls of toilet paper"). On the way to becoming food, some of these fibers are converted into film used for creating rayon, cellophane, and an edible version of cellophane for sausage casing; others go on to become cigarette filters and paint additives. Specialty products made from cellulose fibers find their way into LCD panels, wide-screen, plasma TVs, and non-glare outdoor billboards. Only the purest cellulose is reserved for food-grade gum and used in Twinkies.

When those rolls of "blotter paper" arrive at Hercules Incorporated's Aqualon division, near Williamsburg, Virginia, the only cellulose gum processor in the United States, they are ground up and tossed into a reactor vessel to be cooked in a chemical bath containing lye and sodium monochloroacetate, a pungent, toxic, white petrochemical generally associated with making dyes and herbicides rather than snack food. The resultant mush is washed with water and solvents until it has been transformed into a water-soluble food product known to the pros as sodium carboxymethylcellulose, but thankfully, to the rest of us, as CMC. CMC is not a food you could ever imagine making yourself, or even an ingredient you could imagine using in a recipe, but it is technically food nonetheless.

Dried and ground into a tasteless, odorless fine powder for use by the bakeries, cellulose gum is ready at last to be blended into the mix for Twinkies filling. You better believe that the fifty-pound bags cellulose gum is transported in are well-lined with plastic to keep the CMC dry: its major attribute is that it soaks up water like a sponge.

The Secret Recipe

I once casually asked a Hostess employee point blank for the creamy filling recipe. Instead of the expected formal denial, "I'm not at liberty to disclose such confidential information," or the bracing, "If I told you, I'd have to kill you," I got a great, big, Cheshire cat grin. Nothing more. Perhaps Hostess feels it is its favorite secret, or that while anyone can make a cake, only Hostess can concoct a great creamy filling (with a twenty-five-day shelf life). But while greatness can be deliberated or debated, only cellulose gum can make the creme filling work.

Despite Hostess's secret recipe, most food scientists will tell you that while the main ingredients in the filling are superfine sugar, shortening (oil), corn syrup, water, polysorbate 60, and salt (and certainly not any cream), the key is that old pastry standby, cellulose gum, which can absorb fifteen to an astounding twenty times its own weight in water. A pinch sprinkled on water floats like a jellyfish. A moistened spoonful becomes a clear, gelatinous, slimy glob in a matter of minutes. Intriguingly, though, if left out in the open (as scientifically verified in my office, of course) it dries out in a day or so to leave nothing but a small piece of crisp film (it's a polymer, like latex paint). Air-tight packaging is obviously key.

Cellulose gum hangs on to the water in Twinkies filling, and thus, like so many other ingredients, keeps it slipperier, longer. Its fibers plump the filling up, replacing fat (i.e., real cream) with a moist, glossy, fatlike texture, without contributing a single calorie to the cake because cellulose gum is not digested. Food scientists call it a fat-reducer ingredient. It can be used to reduce oil, butter, or sugar and still keep dressings, icings, and syrups smooth, spreadable, and thick (sample the Slim-Fast Optima™ French Vanilla Shake). It's what helps hold a flavor on the back of your tongue, and, quite literally, helps Twinkies filling to shine.

Cellulose gum also plays a rather magical, if minor, role in the crumb. Food scientists say that the gum "stabilizes" a cake's crumb, or that it "controls staling," which, of course, goes back to the all-important shelf life.

These are the showy accomplishments, but cellulose gum works hard behind the scenes, too. It goes to work early in the cake-baking process, creating an oily smoothness that helps the batter flow properly through the various tanks and pumps that squirt it into the famous finger-cake molds. This means, among other things, that it helps suspend air bubbles in the batter while being crushed by the hundreds of pounds of pressure that are created on the bottom of a two-hundred-gallon batter holding tank. Cellulose gum also captures the pressurized air that is injected into the batter as it enters the continuous mixer right before it hits the oven. You don't have this problem at home, of course, where a whipped batter that weighs mere ounces is poured into molds immediately after being made.

Cellulose gum is not a household item, although its close cousin, pectin, is a popular ingredient for making jams and jellies and is responsible for thickening (and maintaining the suspension of) a Starbucks® Frappuccino®.

Cheap, Nonfattening Food and Osama bin Laden

Totally transparent, tasteless, and versatile, it's obvious why cellulose gum is a popular ingredient found in abundance in your pantry and on your table. It's responsible for the smoothness in McCormick® Au Jus Gravy Mix as well as Swiss Miss® Hot Cocoa Mix, and Starbucks® Low Fat Latte ice cream. To make a low-calorie pancake syrup, you need something viscous to take the place of corn syrup and sugar. Cellulose gum to the rescue! It's the same for many fat-free salad dressings, including Wish-Bone® Fat Free Chunky Blue Cheese.

CMC works in some nonfood products, too, such as bulk laxatives, cosmetics, toothpaste, and that lovely counterpoint to Twinkies, denture adhesives. Cellulose gum is known as a film-former, and helps coat paper, finish smooth textiles, and—I'm not making this up—glaze ceramics. Various versions of cellulose gum are found in at least two hundred different products, including diapers and napkins (for absorbency), drilling fluids (for slipperiness and thickness), and liquid detergents (for a syrupy consistency). All are unlikely cousins to Twinkies creme filling, but are cousins nevertheless.

But cellulose gum is not the only gum with these talents. There are similar gums, each with slightly different gelling, binding, or thickening characteristics, that are often found on ingredient labels and hail from diverse and somewhat exotic sources. Gums may come from trees (locust bean, tree seeds from the Mediterranean, and acacia gum, or gum arabic, from acacia tree sap in the Sahel region of Africa), seaweed (agar, carrageenan, aka Irish moss, and alginates, mostly from the Philippines), pealike plant seeds (guar gum, from India, Pakistan, and the southwestern United States), and bacterial fermentation (xanthan gum, fermented in good old Midwestern corn syrup). Travel to see gum and you'll see the world. Even Osama bin Laden once owned part of an acacia gum firm in Sudan, but was forced to sell out when Sudan booted him in 1996.

Trees and cotton are chopped down, chopped up, soaked, cooked, dried, and chopped and cooked again, all in the name of Twinkies. Former waste products are changed into versatile, natural, and extraordinarily helpful food additives for Twinkies' crumb and filling. Gum is full of surprises. And milk, too, it turns out. Like the crafty few who saw almost limitless potential in cellulose gum, cheese-makers who caused weeds to grow in Wisconsin for years discovered yet another miracle food.

CHAPTER 13

Whey

Whey starts with weeds in Wisconsin.

Watching twenty-pound blocks of mozzarella cheese squeeze out of a stainless steel machine and plop into a bright, pale, yellow-green river that flows through a white fiberglass trough does not exactly stimulate the appetite, but it does evoke curiosity. This is cheese-making, Wisconsin-style. I'm at the biggest cheese factory east of the Mississippi, perhaps the third largest in all the country, to find out how they make whey, the twenty-third ingredient on the Twinkies label.

WHY WHEY?

Sometime in the 1950s—no one seems to have kept track— enterprising local farmers couldn't help but notice the sturdy weeds growing along streams behind cheese-making plants, and somehow realized that the cause of this fecundity was the watery waste spun off at the beginning of the cheese-making process, which was discharged out the back of the plant, and had been since the first big plants were built in the 1800s. Ever resourceful, these farmers started using whey as a natural, low-cost, effective fertilizer; but it wasn't until 1962 that anyone conducted a formal study to confirm that whey, in fact, did facilitate plant growth and might well be safe for human consumption (it came from milk, so this should not have been a stretch). Within ten years, this waste product had become a profitable by-product, and one of the most recent additions to Twinkies' list of master ingredients.

Whey may be good for you—whey is high in minerals (like calcium), lactose (80 percent), and protein (10 to 13 percent)—but that's not why it's used in Twinkies. Sure, it is nutritious in a con-centrated form (creatively named "whey protein concentrate"), but sweet whey is often used in baked goods to aid browning and help develop flavor, something particularly important in a recipe like Twinkie's, which lacks real dairy. The browning occurs as whey's lactose reacts with its protein at conveniently lowish tem-peratures, presumably allowing for a shorter baking time. Pro-cessed food manufacturers like Hostess like dry whey because it minimizes the need for eggs and milk, both of which are costly, difficult to handle, fat-laden, and which spoil. And whey is con-sidered a totally natural ingredient—the processing involves only separating and drying, no chemical reactions—so you can have your cake and eat it, too.

Whey is actually found in your kitchen, in the form of milk, cream, or butter. For years, commercial bakeries used nonfat dried milk to make things like Twinkies before they switched to the more efficient (and less expensive) whey and whey protein concentrate in the 1980s.

Why is whey so popular with bakers of both bread and cakes? Because it helps bind water, slow staling, and keep cakes "moist and fresh" after days or weeks on a store shelf. But bakery prod-ucts only account for about 10 percent of the whey produced. Over half goes into dairy products like yogurt, yogurt bars, cheese products like Kraft® American cheese or Velveeta® cheese sauces, and macaroni and cheese mixes. It is the main ingredient in Kraft's Cheez Whiz® cheese dip as well as the aerosol American cheese product, Easy Cheese®. Whey and whey protein concentrate bind water in processed meats like sausage and hot dogs, add substance to soups, and suggest the "cheese" or "cream" in snacks such as Doritos® and Wise® Sour Cream and Onion Potato Chips. The amount of water retained is a major factor in the way processed foods taste, but not just because of moisture. As whey is baked, its proteins react chemically to create what food scientists call "favorable viscosity" and "heat-setting gel characteristics" (or "gelation"), and what you and I call a smooth texture—just the feeling that Hostess wants you to have when eating a Twinkie.

Better than milk, whey dissolves easily and has only a mild dairy taste, and the way it holds water makes it an excellent emulsifier, fat replacer, and a good source of nonfat dairy solids. As such, it works well in frozen desserts like Good Humor® ice cream bars and Fudgsicles®, or Tollhouse® Mint Brownie Bars. It helps improve and stabilize ice cream's texture, reducing freeze-thaw.

Whey proteins can also be whipped to create a stable foam, making them an important component in chiffon cakes and whipped toppings as well as mochi ice cream balls. That's why whey is found in instant soup, and near the top of the ingredient list in fat-free or low-fat, dairy-accented salad dressings like creamy Italian or blue cheese. Whey adds opacity and viscosity to cream soups, without having to use that perishable (and expensive) cream. As the body-building industry discovered in the 1990s, whey is an excellent protein source with highly efficient muscle-building properties. Whey is now found in nutraceuticals, nutrition bars, sports and nutrition drinks, and infant formula. Because it contains the same proteins as human milk, which has a slightly different protein and lactose content than cow's milk, one of the most exciting possible uses for concentrated whey protein—made by filtering or reacting it on a molecular level—is in developing inexpensive and easily transported protein supplements for starving populations in remote areas of the world. (This could pit Wisconsin against Iowa, the leading soybean producer, on the farm field instead of the football field.) Dairy-based food coating or glaze (like that used on candy) is another promising possible future use—as an alternative to the currently popular shellac (yes, shellac) product.

Whey derivatives also act as bacteriastats and antimicrobial agents in products as diverse as shampoo, acne medicine, toothpaste, cosmetic creams, and chewing gum—possibly even as an oxygen barrier in plastic packaging. But to get here, whey must be processed and concentrated, and that takes big equipment and money.

GREEN RIVER AND STAINLESS VINES

Waupun, Wisconsin—simply the intersection of County Road AA and County Road EE—is in the heart of "the nation's dairy state," full of rich, dark, soft soil, right near the fascinating and enormous Horicon marsh—the largest freshwater cattail marsh in the United States and a designated Globally Important Bird Area. Local bulletin boards are plastered with posters for polka contests and traditional Swiss concerts featuring yards-long alpenhorns. Even the smallest country lanes are paved, in order to allow the dairy trucks smooth and easy access to the farms and dairies (there are sixteen thousand dairy farms in Wisconsin, 99 percent family-owned).

Gleaming, polished, stainless steel milk haulers circulate among the local dairy farms on those nicely paved roads, picking up raw milk daily. Most comes from Holsteins, one of the oldest and most productive dairy breeds in the world. Their drivers develop important long-term relationships with each farmer—no one wants fresh milk to sit around, so timing is critical. The modern Alto Dairy Cooperative sees about eighty tankers a day, each carrying an average of fifty thousand pounds of milk. That's 4 million pounds of milk a day moving through here.

Each cheese-making vat holds about a tanker-load of milk. A starter culture, which contains bacteria that turn the milk sour, is mixed in for fifteen to ninety minutes. Then an enzyme is added to thicken it and encourage coagulation into (solid) curds and (watery) whey, also known as milk serum—the same light yellow-green stuff that sits on top of yogurt that hasn't been stirred in a while. The enzyme, which is the modern replacement of rennet (traditionally scraped off of calves' stomachs), is derived from genetically engineered microbes (bacteria), made by "culture houses," and are the same enzymes that are used for making corn syrups and for brewing lactic acid, two other Twinkie ingredients.

After about two hours, the curds, which look just like white Cheez Doodles® or Styrofoam packing "peanuts," are full of casein and fat, pressed into cheese or sold (fresh only) at the factory store as local, smooth-tasting, fat-laden snacks that squeak as you bite them. (Little Miss Muffet was definitely on to something, I thought, as I ate the delicious curds sitting in my rented Chevy, eschewing a tuffet.) The whey is then siphoned off the top and pumped into the adjoining building. Whey is sometimes labeled as "sweet dairy whey" to differentiate it from acid whey, which is a byproduct of ricotta- or cottage cheese–making. Food companies include the word "dairy" on the ingredient label just to help people who are allergic to dairy products notice the presence of a dairy product.

It takes ten pounds of milk, a bit more than one gallon, to make a pound of cheese, and in those nine leftover pounds are whey solids and a lot of water—94 percent, in fact—so drying it takes some work. The goal is to remove the water and isolate the protein, lactose, and minerals in a usable form. They don't feed any weeds here anymore.

The whey plant is a five-story-high precast concrete box (some of the rooms are actually labeled as tornado shelters) and full of surprises, ranging from small to overwhelming. The first is the sticky doormat just inside the door. Thinking I have stepped in some spoiled spilled milk, I stare dumbly at my gooey feet. My guides, two athletic-looking women, get a good laugh: the mat I've stepped on is designed to remove dirt from shoes. Inside another door, I gingerly step into an unavoidable mound of white foam, thinking once again that I did something bad. The women laugh once more: the foam is disinfectant, sprayed continually on the floor. Cleanliness is clearly paramount here.

The inside of the whey plant can only be likened to an absurd, industrial disco, complete with a hall of long, round mirrors. Filled from floor to ceiling and wall to wall with brilliantly polished two- and four-inch-diameter stainless steel pipes, and shining, human-size conical centrifuges (which spin off butterfat for butter), the area seems paneled in stainless steel. Some of the steel pipes carry whey in and out of various processors, some bring sanitizing products in and out (for constant cleaning of the web), and some simply carry cooling water. The floors are spotless and there is no smell; it is all brilliantly lit so that the place gleams.

The two women hand me off to Joel Denk, Whey Division Manager, who gives me both a physical and academic tour of the plant, where I see that the rest of the whey is first pasteurized and then boiled in a series of forty-foot-tall heat exchangers called effects (the same as those used for sugar and several other Twinkies ingredients), then sent through ten sixty-foot-tall, ten-foot-wide vacuum evaporators that reduce its water content by about half. The watery discharge is boiled at a lower pressure and a lower temperature in each successive evaporator—at one point, the pressure is so low, it boils at only 62°F. It is recirculated as much as a dozen times until it reaches a thick milk-shake consistency, and is then passed through a chilled vat called a crystallizer that resembles an ice cream maker. Here, lactose crystals form so they can easily be removed.

The remaining milk shake is finally sprayed at such high pressure that it is atomized as it shoots into the top of a twenty-five-foot-wide, 60-foot-high, 400°F dryer, one of the largest in the world. It processes twelve thousand pounds of dry whey per hour, twenty-two hours a day. The duct feeding the hot air to the dryer is the size of a hallway, and the blower is a twelve-foot-diameter fan. At the top of the building, it is especially hot, akin to standing right next to a pizza oven. After a few seconds of free-fall, the whey, now an off-white, slightly sticky powder, lands on a conveyor belt, ready for packing and shipping. The daily 4 million pounds of liquid whey has been reduced to about 264,000 pounds, now that the water is gone.

✳

Whey has come a long way from when it was pumped out of cheese plants as so much wasted, watery stuff.

As even better uses for whey are discovered, it's conceivable to imagine that milk output might have to increase to meet the demand, resulting in an excess of milk or cheese. Denk implies that that's why the dairy industry would also love to simply increase the protein in the milk to start with, something that might be done through genetic engineering of cows.

Ultimately, whey's story is wonderfully instructive and, like most food additives, very much a part of the times. A totally natural part of food, it became a separate product by chance thousands of years ago, when cheese-making began with the simple salting and drying of curds. The ancients (Hippocrates, along with Miss Muffet of the sixteenth century—yes, she really existed) enthusiastically drank their whey, and as recently as the nineteenth century,

Swiss spa-goers considered it a health booster, after which whey fell out of favor as a food. It is only within the last few generations that whey has been considered valuable enough to be worth processing. And only most recently did we develop the technology to benefit from whey across the spectrum of food products, from Twinkies to health bars. While it could be argued that it might be simpler to just drink milk and eat yogurt to ingest whey protein, it's hard to argue with progress.

In fact, Twinkies (and most other cakes, too) owe their modern lightness to some ingenious inventors and businessmen who embraced progress in the name of the search for chemical leavening.

CHAPTER 14

Leavenings

R ocks make cakes light and airy.

Believe it or not, the sources of the three chemical leavening ingredients on the Twinkies' label are rocks: phosphate rock, a sodium-rich rock called trona, and calcium-rich limestone. Together, they comprise a strange and active trio. Pure phosphorus bursts into flames when it comes into contact with air. Lime nuggets disintegrate if they are not stored in an airtight container. And almost all sodium bicarbonate, also known as baking soda, is water-soluble and comes from deep mines out in Wyoming.

It's not easy to make the mental adjustment to baking with rocks. It's a pretty big leap to mentally link the humble Twinkie to a mountain-size mine, as well as to accept the rather incongruous fact that leavening for feather-light cakes comes from heavy, dirty, hard substances. So this set of ingredients required a little extra investigation.

Leavening is what makes baked goods rise. You can get it from microbes (yeast), elbow grease (whipping your egg-laden batter full of air), or rocks (chemical baking powder). Without leavening, bread would simply be matzos: no bagels, no buns, no

Twinkies. And while Twinkies are labeled "sponge cake," and sponge cakes are generally leavened by eggs, Twinkies, in order to extend shelf life and reduce expense, contain no fresh eggs, and so require chemical leavening. They also use fat (oil/shortening), making them more of a génoise, in fact, but we won't go there.

Chemical leavening has been sold to the consumer as baking powder in the same basic formula since around 1885, under the familiar brand names and in the familiar small cans of Clabber Girl®, Davis®, and Calumet®. Baking powder is made from sodium bicarbonate (baking soda) and two acid salts, usually monocalcium phosphate and sodium acid pyrophosphate, both of which are found in Twinkies; or sodium aluminum sulfate, found in some brands of baking powder. Add water, and this combination of base and acid fizzes quickly, creating little gas bubbles that get trapped in the batter as it is mixed, which causes the batter to rise. The heat of baking agitates the chemicals once more, causing them to make more gas, hence the term, "double-acting." The theory is simple—combine an acid and a base, get a reaction—but the way to harvest and release gas predictably eluded discovery for ages.

RISING ISSUES

One tends to think of leavening as a common consumer item, but for millennia, leavening was limited to natural, wild yeast. Anyone could leave a primal soup of water, grain, and maybe a little sugar somewhere warm and wait for yeast cells to fall from the air into the fecund mixture. This is how beer-brewing, which predates bread-baking, got started in ancient Sumeria and led to the start of farming and civilization as we know it. Later, cooks learned to keep a "starter" of this type of yeast on the back of a stove for continual use for bread-making, with often delicious but usually inconsistent results. Besides, it was inconvenient. It is hard to keep starter properly, and yeast-raised breads took (and still take) hours to prepare.

Twinkies are a product of the drive to create a modern chemical leavening, part of the modern cultural desire for commercial baked goods. Modern baking experts claim that as far back as when people started eating bread, cooks have been on the lookout for faster, more convenient, and more predictable leavening. This modern drive is based, of course, on the huge consumer and industrial demand that came along with the urbanization and industrialization of society in the 1800s and 1900s, but the impetus dates back even further. While there's evidence that even Renaissance cooks experimented with a tasty powder made of horns, hooves, and leather, it was early American cooks who led the way to find simple leavening.

Colonists first discovered (or learned from the Native Americans, it's not clear) that pearlash—a crude potassium bicarbonate made from wood ashes and normally used for soap and glassmaking—could be added to bread dough to counter the natural sourness of sourdough. (Historians can only guess that this was discovered by accident when some kitchen fire ashes fell into some dough.) Pearlash soon became prized for another effect: the quick rising it produced. By the 1760s it was quite popular among cooks—even then, people wanted things done faster. A revolutionary development in pre-Revolutionary times, the advent of so-called quick breads, like muffins or pancakes or biscuits—so called because without yeast, they do not require any rising time—marked the first use of chemical leavening. (Recipes calling for pearlash appeared in the first American cookbook, Amelia Simmons's *American Cookery*, in 1796.) But using potassium bicarbonate alone didn't work well. Gas tended to be released during mixing (the "bench" phase), before baking, and control was often lost, leading to hit-or-miss results.

The U.S. Patent Office granted only three patents in 1790, its first year of existence. Two of the three related directly to Twinkies (but no, not for Twinkies themselves, as all-American as they might be). One concerned the manufacture of pearlash, the precursor of baking powder, and the other was for automated flour-milling machinery, which led to fine, white flour. Both are evidence of the importance of our cultural drive for improved cake-baking.

Around 1802, Oliver Evans, the American inventor of one of the first steam-operated vehicles as well as the high-pressure steam engine, opened the first steam-powered flour mill, in Delaware, producing lighter, finer flour than was ever possible before (while Scottish engineer James Watt had built the first one in England in 1780, American relations with the Brits were a bit troubled just then, putting a damper on transatlantic commerce). In the early 1800s, as the country became more developed, educated, and urbanized, Americans were focusing a lot of research on household chemistry. Ways to achieve convenience and lightness in baking with the newly available finer flour naturally followed.

But there was a problem with the early baking powders: acid. Sour milk isn't the most reliable ingredient, it seems, and other alternative acid sources such as lemon juice, vinegar, or tartaric acid (derived from cream of tartar, scraped from the sides of wine barrels, and imported from Italy and France's wine-making regions) tasted pretty bad or were too expensive to be used widely. Finally, no available acid source could be premixed with the dry base (whether pearlash or sodium bicarbonate) without it reacting prematurely.

The big breakthrough—the perfection of modern baking powder—came in 1859, from none other than Harvard University.

BUBBLES AND THE COUNT

Eben Norton Horsford was a chemistry professor at Harvard for sixteen years, from 1847 to 1863, where he had occupied the Rumford Chair of the Application of Science to the Useful Arts, a Harvard chemistry professorship endowed in 1814 by Benjamin Thompson, an American inventor and scientist. (Thompson was one of the discoverers of the law of conservation of energy and applied it to the famous Rumford fireplace, a state-of-the-art heating appliance of the 1790s. Later, he was given the honorary title of "Count Rumford" because he worked for the Bavarian government for a long time.) The chair was dedicated to those scientists who showed exceptional achievements in "the useful domestic arts," what we might have called home economics. Not only did Horsford's invention lead to a company that exists still, but the product he invented is essential to anyone who calls him or herself a cook (a professional or amateur), and has been since 1859. Twinkies, for one thing, could never have existed without him. Thank you, Harvard.

After years of experimenting with hundreds of acid sources in Cambridge and Germany, Horsford found that by saturating animal bones from nearby slaughterhouses in sulfuric acid, he could manufacture a crude form of monocalcium phosphate that could be dried into a powder and mixed with sodium bicarbonate to create a dry chemical leavening that fizzed when wet. But he still faced some challenges. Phosphoric acid alone meant that most of the leavening action was brought on by moisture, so he worked to refine the monocalcium phosphate for more consistent and better-tasting results. The 1885 discovery of a sodium acid phosphate that gave off gas in response to heat, not water, led to its inclusion in the mix, for a "secondary action"—the action that gave us the term "double-acting." Now, when Horsford mixed it with sodium bicarbonate, he had the first phosphate-based, stable, reliable, affordable baking powder, which he packaged as Rumford®, in honor of the great Count, whose beribboned, ponytailed cameo still graces the label on cans today. Horsford's success was so significant that the original Rumford, Rhode Island, site of his business, Rumford Chemical Works, has now been designated by the American Chemical Society a National Historic Chemical Landmark, complete with a museum (run by the East Providence Historical Society) of baking soda–related paraphernalia, such as cookbooks, kitchen tools (given away as premiums), company photographs, patent records, and original cans. The company was eventually sold to Clabber Girl, which sometime in the 1960s moved Horsford's laboratory intact to Terre Haute, Indiana, where it is now a small museum at Rumford's current corporate headquarters, one of the city's fine attractions and further testimony to Horsford's success.

Rumford Baking Powder was one of the world's first convenience foods to be offered to the modern housewife, though it met with a little resistance. Some associated it with poor, lazy, or unfeminine wives, who, it was felt, should take no shortcuts with their breads. On the other hand, when Louis Pasteur revealed the presence of microbes to the public, old-fashioned, natural yeast instantly seemed unappealing. The clean, white, chemical powder suddenly became a popular alternative in the consumer's new and energetic quest for cleanliness. It didn't hurt that its chemicals were already found in the human body, either.

Although other scientists developed baking powder at about the same time in England and in Germany, it was Horsford who helped usher in the glorious concept of truly American cooking by making possible such chemically leavened items as blueberry muffins, biscuits, cake mixes, and, of course, Twinkies.

But whether an industrial or consumer product, leavening is made from the same basic recipe today, often with a touch of cornstarch or calcium sulfate (both of which are Twinkies ingredients) to improve shelf life or control humidity. And all the major brands boast old-fashioned-looking logos and labels, a testimony to legendary brand loyalty among home cooks. (Clabber Girl's dates back to 1899, though the girl on the label is modern, by comparison, having arrived in 1923. Rumford has the oldest consumer product label found in grocery stores, dating back to the 1860s.)[10]

The big bakeries have to mix their own baking powder to meet their more demanding manufacturing conditions, usually requiring more secondary action to closely control the rising in the oven. So they often buy the three ingredients—sodium bicarbonate, monocalcium phosphate, and sodium acid pyrophosphate—directly from their manufacturers, such as FMC in Green River, Wyoming, and Innophos in Chicago, Illinois. In order to make all that gas, you need rocks, and to find out where these gas-producing rocks come from calls for a trip out West. An underground trip, it turns out.

---

10. The late 1800s was a period of newly improved commerce and communication, some sophisticated (railroads, newspapers, telegraph) and some not (snake oil and other creative traveling salesmen). This was fertile ground for the wild claims and major ad campaigns of early baking powders—Clabber Girl® and Davis®, as well as Oetker and Kraft's Calumet® Baking Powder, all still alive and competing today, even if (curiously) Rumford®, Clabber Girl®, and Davis® are now all made by the same company—including spurious assertions that competitors' powders, among the first chemicals sold as convenience food, were made with poison. This led to the demand for honesty in packaging, which in turn led to the 1905 ingredient labeling laws that formed the basis for the labels we have today—and the inspiration for this book.

CHAPTER 15

Baking Soda

Hurtling 1,600 feet downward at a windy 450 feet per minute in an open-mesh steel cage the size of a double garage, I'm risking my life—or, at least, my sanity—to see where the raw ingredient shared by two of the leavening ingredients on the Twinkies label comes from. Leavening makes things go up, but to see it I'm going down—way down.

I'm wearing earplugs, amplifying the machinery's rumbling and clanging sounds inside my head, along with a blinding miner's lamp on my hard hat that makes for constantly moving shadows. My knees are a little weak with fright and the big, tough-looking miners standing around me are not reassuring, even if I could hear them through my earplugs and over the roar of the wind and the machinery. I am having trouble connecting this experience with the ubiquitous little yellow box of baking soda that sits in so many kitchen cabinets and refrigerators around the world.

I'm also wearing safety glasses, brand-new cotton gloves, and a wide tool belt with a very heavy battery for my headlamp ("Good for sixteen hours!" my host reassures me), as well as a canteen-size emergency self-rescue carbon monoxide breathing kit in case of fire. I've also been given a dust mask ("just in case") and a course in mine safety for which I am presented with an official U.S. Department of Labor Certificate of Training. All this just to see where an unassuming kitchen staple comes from?

Tim Davis, a Senior Mining Engineer with FMC Corporation and my guide, tells me to avoid looking him or others in the face because the bright miner's lamp on my helmet will blind them. The word is, never look a miner in the eye. So we all affect a slightly bashful stance as we descend, painting the floor with pools of light as we head down into raw baking soda.

Finding Wyoming

Green River, Wyoming, a region of brown earth and white alkali flats, sits atop the world's largest and purest trona deposit, which is not very impressive to most people because they have never heard of it. Trona was discovered in 1938, almost by accident when Mountain Fuel Supply, a company then based in Ohio (and now part of the much larger Questar natural gas company), drilled a wildcat exploratory oil well in this mineral-rich area along the Oregon Trail. Instead of oil, they found soft, brown, layered stone. A sample was sent to the U.S. Geological Survey office in Washington, D.C., where it sat, ignored, for more than a year.

When the agency finally got around to analyzing it, the geologists found that it was a sedimentary rock made largely of pure sodium sesquicarbonate, which is easily cooked into sodium carbonate, commonly known as soda ash. Soda ash is the basic chemical ingredient in glass and soap, its most common and ancient uses (about half of the soda ash produced goes into glass); it is also widely used in hundreds of essential chemical products including detergents and water softeners. And it is where the "sodium" in sodium bicarbonate—baking soda—comes from, as well as the sodium in the other baking powder ingredient, sodium acid pyrophosphate. (It is a common source of sodium for sodium stearoyl lactylate, too, an unrelated Twinkies additive.) So soda ash finds its way, indirectly, into much of what we eat, which is pretty alarming, considering it is also the primary component of glass and soap.

FMC Corporation, one of the world's larger chemical companies, opened the world's first and now largest trona mine and processing complex here in 1952. Other companies, such as Church & Dwight (makers of Arm & Hammer® Baking Soda), also access the thousand-square-mile ore patch, thanks in part to antitrust laws that force them to share. Underground, their mines come as close as within one hundred feet of each other. Today, even though companies in Ohio and New York also make bicarb (often for "store" brands), almost all American soda ash, the main ingredient in sodium bicarbonate, comes from here.

This area is vast, flat, and photogenic, dotted with sagebrush and shrubs. Buttes and ridges puncture the horizon, while antelope roam alongside the highway. FMC's No. 8 Shaft is a group of several two-story, plain brown and tan corrugated steel office buildings with a modest three-story tower behind them. It stands in the center of nothing, but also not far from Route 80 and its New Jersey–like traffic. Outside, there is a little feeder for the wild rabbits of the area. It is an oasis in the desert, an island in the ocean.

The entry to the mine is not much more than a locker room and a big freight elevator (called a hoist here), complete with an airlock, bright, full-size traffic lights, and warning signs that look like they belong over a highway exit. The trophy case is full of awards for mine rescue team operations rather than bowling league trophies or displays of clients' products, giving a visitor pause.

After getting in the hoist cage, it's a free fall for what feels like an eternity. It is not like the subway or a skyscraper express elevator at all, unless, perhaps, in combination. Imagine an express subway train on a vertical track with excruciatingly long pauses between stations. (Even the eighty-floor express elevator to New York City's Empire State Building observation deck takes only fifty seconds. This so-called elevator takes five minutes and travels more than twice as far.)

Arriving at the bottom, we enter a three-story-high vault full of mining equipment, and my guide commandeers one of the several old, doorless, windowless, white diesel CJ7 Jeeps. Sixteen hundred feet below the surface of the earth, we drive through miles of old tunnels at a good fifteen miles per hour for half an hour in order to reach the active mining face. We cross paths with no one, despite crossing other tunnels every 125 feet. This place contains a city's worth of roadway (literally more than four thousand miles, four times more than San Francisco's streets) in tunnels fifteen feet wide and nine feet high—the thickness of the seam of ore that they are mining—and it covers an area almost forty miles square. This grid of activity has been constructed since 1952, under the quiet desert plain above. And while it is sobering to realize that these endless roadways belong solely to FMC, only one of four mining companies in this patch, or seam or bed, of ore, it is even more amazing to realize that where we are driving was once filled with solid rock, a mineral that has since been dug out, removed, and used to make glass and chemicals and thousands of other different products.

This stuff may be used to make food, but it just looks like rock to me. To say that it does not suggest Twinkies—or any other food product—in the least is the biggest understatement one could make.

Driving through dark tunnels in an open Jeep is so unnerving that as we hurtle along I have to force myself to relax my white-knuckled grip. My right hand is wrapped around a five-foot-long steel crowbar that Tim tells me later is used to pry any pieces of trona that are left dangling from the ceiling; my left hand is tight around a sturdy canvas strap that I realize, once we stop, is no safety handle—it is only my camera bag.

At the mining face, a giant, ten-foot-diameter, three-layered claw of a cutting wheel with dozens of sharp points carves out trona at the rather astounding rate of 1,200 tons per hour, stopping only for periodic maintenance. It is mounted on heavy machinery the size of a tank, all of which was brought into the mine disassembled and reconstructed on the spot. It fills the space, and would be totally at home in a special-effects movie.

A long, solid steel conveyor spans the few hundred feet of the floor from the cutting machine to the entrance. No belt here—the broken rock drops onto the steel and is pushed along by arms that move continuously on the shiny steel track. Occasionally, the miners whack some oversize chunks with a shovel or a sledgehammer, the ore being soft enough to respond. The gale of ventilating air flaps my heavy canvas safety equipment belt vigorously. The dust is nontoxic, but as an added bonus, the miners needn't worry about acid indigestion. This is medicine as well as food.

What's most intriguing about this underground landscape is what's missing: the close walls ("pillars" in mine-speak) holding up the ground above, forming tunnels. Here, the roof, 750 feet long and about twenty feet wide, is held up only temporarily by a row of 135, C-shaped, computer-operated, hydraulic steel supports, like forklifts on steroids (putting out 750 tons of pressure each), lined up right next to one another in a long row of sheer, ten-foot-tall strength. The top arms are about fourteen feet long, the feet about eight and a half, and each unit is five or six feet wide. As the digging progresses, the whole shebang is moved along: the digger, the conveyor, and the self-powered supports, a few at a time, thirty-two inches for each cut. The ceiling of shale behind the cut is simply allowed to collapse. This is supposedly safe, but when a chip drops and bangs onto my hard hat, I jump about a foot.

However safe this might be, the wall creaks and cracks continuously. It even splashes, as big chunks of rock split and fall off, contrasting with the otherwise eerie underground silence. My engineer guide explains that this is good rock mechanics. You take out tons of rock, the land above presses down, the rock cracks. "You don't want stress to build up," says Tim. "It has to be relieved, periodically, in small amounts, just like with us," otherwise it might just all cave in.

The material is coaxed along the steel conveyor, into a small crusher, and onto the eight-mile-long rubber conveyor belt for the trip to the soda ash plant, our next destination, where it will emerge into a neat pile.

A few prairie dogs dart in front of my car, narrowly escaping with their lives, as I drive to the plant. In fact, I'm driving over the very spot I was under all morning, looking for where this Twinkie ingredient comes from. The next step is to make it into some useful things, like soda ash and sodium bicarbonate. The soda processing plant must be the whitest plant in the world, and it hasn't snowed for weeks. All the buildings and machinery are dusted with trona or soda ash, contrasting beautifully with the dark brown, vast, open, classic western landscape. Sagebrush and soda.

The Guillotine, the Arm, and the Hammer

Some food sources are planted in the spring and harvested in the fall. This one was planted 50 to 60 million years ago, and has been constantly harvested since 1952. Lake Gosiute, an eight-thousand-square-mile, Eocene epoch subtropical lake, filled and evaporated repeatedly, and trona formed thanks to the introduction of considerable amounts of carbon dioxide (either from de-caying plants and animals or from hydrothermal activity—no one knows). This left behind a rock layer of ancient marine deposits and 150 billion tons of trona in a dozen seams sandwiched between layers of shale and sandstone that came to be known as the Green River Basin.

Nowhere else in the world is there anything quite like this deposit, a thousand square miles of trona. Though only about a third of it is recoverable, there is enough for world demand for more than four thousand years to come (based only on current mining techniques, that figure is reduced considerably and open to debate). FMC alone processes nearly 7 million tons each year into soda ash; all the mining companies together have the capacity to remove about 15 million tons each year.

But the stats don't tell the whole story. Why is this rock product called soda? Where did we get soda ash before these Green River mines started in the 1950s? And, finally, the fundamental question: how and why did we begin eating this particular rock, putting it into bread, muffins, and, of course, Twinkies?

Soda ash is all about sodium. The term "soda" denotes something that contains sodium (sodium carbonate is also known as sal soda and washing soda). For thousands of years going back to ancient Egypt, crude soda, whether for glass or mummy-making, was made from plant ashes, notably seaweed and trees, giving it the common name soda ash. People simply burnt vegetable matter and then poured water over the ashes to leach out the soda. Early American colonists cut enormous quantities of trees to make soda ash for soap-making and glass-making. They were so productive that they exported eight thousand tons to Europe in 1792 (this was mostly potassium carbonate, or pearlash, baking soda's predecessor). It is possible that more trees were cut for chemicals than for use as fuel; certainly that is what deforested much of Europe and England. Another source that fell into political disfavor was Spanish barilla, a bushy plant that grows in coastal salt marshes. In addition to a political desire to cut dependence on American exports, this deforestation, coupled with increasing demand, is what drove the Europeans to try to develop an industrial source of soda ash.

In 1783, King Louis XVI asked the French Academy of Science to offer a prize of 100,000 francs—probably worth close to three-quarters of a million of today's dollars—to anyone who could develop such a process. In response to that, a Frenchman named Nicolas Leblanc managed to create the modern, artificial source of soda ash, the predecessor source to Green River, but he was unable to capitalize and build plants due to what might be described as acute political problems (among other things, his principal investor was guillotined).

Leblanc had designed a two-step process that called for mixing sea salt and sulfuric acid, and then heating the resulting sodium sulfate with charcoal and limestone. Unfortunately, with these plants, a lot of hydrochloric acid and CO_2 went up the smokestacks (acid rain is nothing new), more hydrochloric acid polluted streams, and copious amounts of black ash and partially burnt coal dumped in surrounding areas polluted the land. England, which had embraced this process, became both the leading chemical producer in the world and one of the first countries to pass an antipollution law, the 1863 Alkali Act. Because of the pollution, the Leblanc process became unpopular just as the product was becoming more in demand, especially by American cooks. This was thanks to a couple of fellows, Church and Dwight, whose product had a little logo that you might recall seeing from time to time: the arm and hammer.

In the 1830s, Dr. Austin Church perfected a way of making inexpensive sodium bicarbonate by cooking expensive English artificial soda ash over coal fires for three weeks at a time, a process that produced what they called salaratus ("aerated salt"). In 1846, he and his brother-in-law, John Dwight, began selling small, retail bags of salaratus—the first baking soda—with great success, in large part due to the fact they now had not only a superior, consistent product, but one that sold in 1850 for pennies a pound versus something that had previously cost on the order of $1.25 a pound. Their current little yellow package still carries the 1846 date, though their claim of "natural" is a bit of a stretch.

Church and Dwight continued to search for a more efficient process in order to meet increased demand. Serendipitously, the first synthetic sodium carbonate plant opened in the United States during this period. The process, developed in 1861 by Belgian scientists Ernest and Alfred Solvay, used a chemical reaction (originally reacting salt with ammonia and limestone, later just using ammonia and coal) that created impure sodium bicarbonate as an intermediate step in the process to make artificial sodium carbonate, or soda ash, which has always been more in demand. Until the Green River mines became operational in the early 1950s, all of our sodium bicarbonate was made using the Solvay process. Now, none of the U.S. soda ash is made this way, but the Solvay process still serves the rest of the world.

Still, some elements of the original product remain unchanged, especially its famous logo. When Dr. Church's son, James, joined the business in 1867, he brought along the logo of the Brooklyn mustard and spice business, Vulcan Spice Mills, where he had been working, despite its apparent lack of connection to baking soda. It depicted the arm and hammer of Vulcan, the Roman god of fire and metalworking, the very same logo Church & Dwight still uses today for its brand, Arm & Hammer®.

TOWER OF BUBBLE

The newly mined trona, at the end of its eight-mile underground conveyor belt, is carried up and spewed onto one of many three-story-high piles next to the soda ash plant. Long, angled, white conveyors, looking like elevated subway tracks, connect several groups of buildings. Each building makes slightly different versions of soda, mostly by dissolving it and then concentrating and drying it to both purify it and to create crystals of a desired size and shape, much like a sugar or salt plant. FMC alone has ten plants here; our destination is the sesquicarbonate, or "sesqui" plant that makes the sodium carbonate that gets processed into sodium *bi*carbonate. White icicles dangle off roofs and hissing valves, suggesting dainty gingerbread houses. The icicles, while not edible, are not toxic. They better not be—after all, much of this stuff goes into our food.

Some of the pipes, carrying six thousand gallons of sesqui slurry per minute, lead to the nearby sodium bicarbonate (or "bicarb") plant, where the plain sodium carbonate will be purified and given some more carbon to become sodium bicarbonate—baking soda, one of the three components of baking powder—in a matter of hours, a day or so after it was raw ore.

Two things welcome you as you enter FMC's bicarb plant headquarters: an informal glass display case in the entry hall that holds dozens of boxes of Little Debbie cakes (it is nice to see an ingredient in its final form not far from its raw source); and the friendly smile of Glenda Thomas, the chemical engineer who runs this place.

The first stop on the plant tour is the small, plain pipe where the soda ash slurry, bicarb's raw material, enters the building. The pipe seems inconsequential, not even a foot in diameter, for a plant that can make seventy thousand tons of bicarb a year. Thomas opens a test hole in a big pipe and takes out a cupful from the torrent to examine. It feels slippery and grainy, a soapy salt solution—a welcome, sensual surprise because so much of the processed materials are in fact hidden in the pipes and ovens and myriad stainless steel devices.

Giant cone-bottomed hoppers fill the room, suspended way above the floor. When viewed from underneath, they look like missiles stored in launch readiness. After a climb to the top of the seven-story carbonation tower, the central and most important point in the process, we can see the actual carbonation take place, transforming this stuff that was just mined into a gold mine of a food product. It simply takes lots of gas, yet another Western resource.

Carbon dioxide comes in via truck from one of a few nearby processors, such as ExxonMobil's Shute Creek natural gas facility, a site that includes hundreds of natural gas wells that are no more than pipes sticking out of the ground with valves on them. ExxonMobil separates the natural gas out and pipes the rest, the CO_2, to a processor that cleans out the remaining methane and sulfur, compresses it, liquefies it, and trucks it over to FMC.

It is hard not to think of this towering tank as a giant seltzer bottle. The CO_2 bubbles up, almost boiling, in a soup of sodium carbonate and water. Local gas and rock are mixed here to make one of the most well-known and widely used household chemicals in the world. From Wyoming to your teeth, your cupboard, your fridge, your cake. And your Twinkie.

A few more ladders and catwalks lead to the "dry" side. The liquid enters the dry side through big pipes and is sent floating down an eight-story cylinder of hot air. Now looking more like moist gravel, it is further dried, cooled, and screened for various crystal sizes in a series of rather compact boxes. Different crystal sizes are desired for various uses: big for animal feed (the most common use—because corn-fed cattle get indigestion of sorts, seeing as they are natural grass eaters, not grain eaters); small for water softening. The crystal size influences the rate of the chemical leavening reaction, too. Every aspect has to be just right so that when wetted and reacted with the phosphoric acid salts in baking powder (or the vinegar in your kitchen), the bicarb releases the carbon dioxide it just picked up here. It all balances out.

We make our way to the end of the production line, and once again Thomas opens a pipe to check out the flow, but this time she scoops out and proudly pours some still-warm, absolutely freshly processed sodium bicarbonate, soft and smoother than talcum powder, onto my hands. I taste it, waiting for the rush, the revelation that every foodie gets from tasting food at its freshest, at its source—the milk drunk while standing by the cow, the wine sampled at the winery—and I am not disappointed. It is the freshest, best-tasting bicarb of soda I have ever had. It is hard to get a sense of terroir that this taste conveys, the taste of the local climate and soil, as this is not fine wine. And, in fact, it is very, very hard to imagine this as having been a rock or a gas, underground and nearby, only days earlier, yet here I am eating it. What's more, this rock powder needs to be mixed with some more powders made from rocks in order to make baking powder. And at least one of them comes from yet another mine just a few miles away.

CHAPTER 16

Phosphates: Sodium Acid Pyrophosphate and Monocalcium Phosphate

As I begin walking across the parking lot behind my historic hotel in Soda Springs, Idaho, a loud whoosh stops me in my tracks. I whip around to see a geyser of carbonated water shooting up a hundred feet and splashing lazily back onto the red-orange-yellow bed of dried minerals in the adjacent lot. There is no shortage of "soda" (as the locals call it)—a reminder of the geologic treasure underground out West.

I'm here to see where another mineral, phosphorus, comes from—the source for phosphoric acid, the stuff that eventually makes the "phosphate" in monocalcium phosphate (MCP) and the "acid" as well as the "phosphate" in sodium acid pyrophosphate (SAPP), the two remaining ingredients that join baking *soda* to make up baking *powder*, or chemical leavening, the very incarnation of modern baking. What that means is that I'm on a trip to see where some rocks we eat come from.

The way it works is this: phosphoric acid is mixed with two bases, limestone and sodium carbonate, to make two new chemicals—and, voilà, baking powder. When baking powder, this mixture of ground-up rocks, is wetted and heated, such as in making, say, Twinkies, the acid and bases react (just like the vinegar and baking soda experiment of your childhood), to create nice little gas bubbles that make cakes like Twinkies so light and airy. As exciting as that is, though, nothing is quite as dramatic as wrenching elemental phosphorus from the earth in order to kick-start the whole process.

Acid Rock

Phosphorus is the source of some of the most common chemicals used in everyday life. It is one of the seven elements necessary for life, and the atomic bonder of the amino acid ladder rungs in DNA (the phosphorus pros showing me around like to joke, "Phosphorus is what holds your genes up!"). It's also what puts the glow in tracer bullets and causes artillery shells to explode, because it bursts into flame when it makes contact with air. So it does seem odd that some Twinkie ingredients are made from it.

Baking powder is only one of the more common uses for food-grade phosphoric acid, which is used in hundreds of ways (among them: setting jam, jelly, and chocolate pudding; gelling processed seafood like surimi [sea legs]; preserving meat in sausage; refining sugar, emulsifying processed cheese, cleaning poultry), and much of it is used as the soft-drink ingredient that gives colas their distinctive tanginess. Phosphoric acid is actually one of the few individual ingredients listed on the Coca-Cola® label, right between "caramel color" and "natural flavors." Surprisingly, though, it is not a major ingredient—less than 1 percent in most food products, used sparingly, much like citric and acetic acids. Industrial uses range from fertilizers to fire retardants to water purification; naval jelly is one form familiar to handypersons as a rust remover. Phosphoric acid does seem like an unlikely food ingredient, especially in something as delicate as cake. It is even harder to believe that it starts out as soft rock.

Dirt versus German Nuns' Urine

The mine of the flammable rock is about eighteen miles up the highway and a few thousand feet higher than Soda Springs, tucked amid softly rounded hills dotted with pockets of trees that form the western edge of the Rockies. Barley fields carpet the valley.

A couple of mining engineers drive me into Monsanto's Enoch Valley Mine, where our sizable Chevy Suburban feels minuscule dodging the huge eighty-five and hundred-ton Caterpillar 777B and 777D trucks that are speeding by, dumping ore, shale, and soil. By dodging, I mean that the engineers in the car recognize that not only do the big monster vehicles have the right-of-way, they have the ability to crush us without even noticing. The car is quiet as we swivel our heads with tense concentration, on the lookout for the oncoming vehicles as we make our way into the 1,800-foot-long and 350-foot-deep pit. The pit is about 1,000 feet wide. The wheels on these ore trucks are so large that I don't even reach the top of the wheel rim when I stand next to one, boots and hard hat included, and I'm close to six feet tall. The ladder for the driver has three steps just to get onto the bumper, and two more, larger ladders to get from there to the cab.

Two big scooper machines, one looking like a regular front loader on steroids, the other a giant crane, are digging and dumping dark dirt into the trucks at a furious pace. The scoops (the buckets) are so big that at over twenty tons each scoop, they fill the trucks in four dumps. A minute or two later, the trucks are rushing off again. The pit is a scene of constant motion that fairly sings, "time is money."

"This is it," says David Carpenter, exploration geologist and one of the mining engineers, proudly pointing at my feet. All I see is dirt. I've traveled to the far reaches of the West to see one of the most exotic minerals around, and, now that I'm here, I'm a bit let down to realize that phosphate ore, which is a soft rock, looks remarkably like plain old black dirt. It crumbles easily when you pick at it—or run at it with a bulldozer the size of a small house. It is called calcium fluorapatite, a fancy name for calcified tropical sea creatures and plants, Pleistocene-era plankton, among others, forced near the surface during the basin and range formation period. The miners call it just plain apatite. I resist the urge to ask them if it is *bon*.

Thirty percent of the nation's phosphate reserves are found here, in what's known as the Western Phosphate Field, within a hundred-mile radius of Soda Springs, Idaho. It was discovered by Wild West gold miners in 1889. The current annual output is more than 6 million tons, divided between fertilizer factories and the big "thermal" phosphorus plant down the road. (The reserves should last well into the 3000s.) It wasn't always mined this way, though. This is a modern source, not the original source of phosphorus, the one where phosphorus was discovered.

Back in the mid-1600s, while amateur German alchemist Henning Brand was a medic in the German army (presumably during the Thirty Years' War), he got the idea from watching the life ooze out of mortally wounded soldiers that the "stuff" of life must be in the liquids of the body. He thought blood research, though common, was "of the devil," so he chose to look at other body fluids, which led him to experiment with urine. (Yes, urine.) In search of the purest, holiest urine he could find, he convinced some nuns near Hamburg to collect and donate their urine, which he then distilled. In 1669, after years of experimenting, he managed to boil the urine in the absence of air down to a ball of waxy goop that either burnt up immediately or glowed, depending on the purity of the "ore." Legend has it that he took a glowing, burning ball into his bed to see if he could soak up some life from it as he slept, but all that happened is that his bedclothes caught fire and he suffered some serious burns. Such an ignominious result for the first positively known discoverer of an element.

Arc Furnaces and Attack Tanks

As difficult as it may be to refine ore, it does seem to be an improvement over urine.

The Monsanto phosphate plant where the trucks deliver the ore is located a few minutes outside of Soda Springs, Idaho, across a much-used freight track where long tank-car chains rumble along, day and night. The plant, at the end of a mile-long conveyor belt, is surrounded by several thirty- or forty-foot-high piles of raw ingredients—a few perfect jet-black cones of coke (pure carbon from cooked coal) and a few similar but light sand-colored cones of silica (quartz). The ore is a longer but lower pile of what looks like a highway ramp construction site, because it just looks like dirt. Coke, silica, and ore: the basic urine-free phosphorus recipe for Twinkies leavening.

The immense mineral wealth of Wyoming and Idaho make this the ideal location for the plant. The coke, silica, and power (coal-generated) come from nearby mines. Railroads crisscross the entire region, as does the Oregon Trail. This is the industrial heartland, although signs along the highway proclaim it the "Barley Capital of the World."

This elemental phosphorus plant is the last and only one in North America, partly due to the cost of electricity (which is free in some foreign countries, an upsetting fact for this plant's owners) and partly due to the environmental concerns triggered by its toxic discharge (another company's plant, which closed in 2001, is now a Superfund site, thanks to elevated levels of arsenic and other pollutants found in local groundwater). This whole process may soon be rendered obsolete by a newer, technologically advanced "wet process" phosphoric acid–making technique. But this process is amazing to behold.

The plant is so big that I have to drive almost a mile to reach the back, where the ore is baked and purified. It rolls through a rotating kiln, twenty feet in diameter and 325 feet long, that bakes it at 2,500°F—so hot that the rock turns into little bumpy stone bits called nodules. The kiln is so massive that observing it from nearby is like watching a football field rotate. It is here that the phosphate ore begins to shed its dirtness and edge toward elemental pureness.

The nodules drop onto one of the country's biggest conveyor belts, after which it ascends to the top of the electric arc furnaces (at nine stories high, the world's largest) and tumble along with a precisely measured, gravelly mixture of coke and silica from the piles outside—two more rocks for leavening, but these we don't eat (they just act as catalysts). Another cooking session begins—this one even hotter. A lot hotter.

As I leave the bright sunshine outside to enter the dark, blackened furnace area, Steve Ahmann, the furnace supervisor, puts on his wraparound sunglasses (and earplugs), which serves as a warning that I'm about to see something spectacular. A skinny young worker with thick, dark goggles and enormous, heat-shielding gloves is tending a magazine-size access hole about halfway up the thick-walled furnace that reveals a sun-like inferno. He is energetically scraping and pushing the melted mass inside with fifteen-foot-long poles, manipulating them through the tiny window, sending off goopy by-products (including vanadium, which is sold to steelmakers). "This job is a rite of passage," Ahmann says. Indeed, a kid straight out of engineering school would do well to work in this Hades awhile, to witness the chemical reaction firsthand, to develop an appreciation for real heat. At these temperatures—11,000°F, close to that of the sun's surface, and just what it takes to melt any and all known materials—the chemicals release their bonds and a plasma forms. Here, rock is instantaneously liquefied in the name of baking powder.

No oxygen is admitted to the oven, so the phosphorus doesn't burn. It escapes out the top as gas in a maze of tubes and scaffolding that gleams in the intense mountain sunlight. As it cools down into a precious, honeylike liquid, it is sent through airtight pipes into waiting railroad tank cars where it is kept from bursting into flames by a protective blanket of water. The railroad cars stay parked for a while to allow for the liquid to cool down to its "freezing" point (about 140°F) so it will solidify, making it safer to transport.

In the nearby quality control lab, technicians proudly display their recent take: a collection of beakers with an inch or two of what looks like dark yellow wax on the bottom, covered by a few inches of water. These beakers sit in a large picnic cooler—which no one gets near unless they are wearing face masks and gloves, as the slightest exposure to air could cause it to burst into flames. Dangerous stuff, this food ingredient. Security here is tight, because pure phosphorus is worth thousands of dollars an ounce on the street, one tech says, stemming from the fact that it is a helpful part of meth production. However, he adds with a grin, if anyone did steal some, the culprit would probably be found at the local emergency room within hours, covered with burns.

The lab techs are not about to sacrifice any of their precious liquid just to show a visitor how flammable it actually is. For that, a burly engineer on a bridge over the railroad tank cars dons a massive, silver, asbestos suit, complete with cylindrical helmet. Looking like a National Geographic volcanologist and playing the Soda Springs, Idaho, version of a vintner sampling a barrel of his wine, he waddles out over the railcar, where a feather of steam is wafting temptingly out of the manhole-like opening, while I peek out nervously from behind a thick steel panel where I have been directed to hide. He dips a narrow siphon tube down through the protective layer of water and lifts it way up, allowing the pure phosphorus to stream back into the tank. It starts by pouring, looking and acting just like water, and after six inches it is flaming.

Indeed, this is what innocuous, everyday baking powder is made of, but most of this elemental phosphorus is used to make acid for Monsanto's Roundup®, the most common herbicide in the world (the one that Monsanto's genetically modified corn and soybean plants resist). Trainloads are headed to Innophos's Nashville, Tennessee, plant to be processed into phosphoric acid in what they call the thermal process. There, this elemental phosphorus is burned in huge towers and the resulting smoke/gas is sprayed with water to make phosphoric acid. It is as close to pure as anything can be.

Phosphoric acid can also be made directly from North Carolinian or Moroccan ore with the newer and more common "wet process" that became popularized worldwide in the 1990s. At Innophos's Geismar, Louisiana, acid plant, phosphate rock, which is loaded with calcium, is reacted with sulfuric acid to form "green" phosphoric acid and calcium sulfate, after which the calcium sulfate (aka gypsum, used to make common plaster) is removed. The ability to filter and purify this acid enough to use in food is big news, a technological leap that only recently occurred and is likely, due to increased costs and environmental concerns, to become the only way we get phosphoric acid in the future.

Tellingly, the big tank used for the reaction is called the attack tank. When I ask a plant manager at another plant if he can sell the calcium sulfate, he mentions that, no, the stuff from his plant is "just a little bit radioactive, thanks to some uranium that happens to be in the ore. We just bury it back in the mines." That's much better than using it to make radioactive wallboard (only pure, mined calcium sulfate is used in food like Twinkies). One plant alone sends 250,000 pounds a year of fresh, pure phosphoric acid to food and chemical plants around the country.

But no matter the type of acid, it is not yet ready for Twinkies' baking powder. For starters, it is still a liquid. It will be transformed into a tame, safe, white powder in Chicago at Innophos's phosphate plant. But two other ingredients need to get there, too: lime and sodium carbonate.

Always Keep Your Rocks from Starting Fires

Limestone is mined from caves dug into the side of rolling hills in a gentler landscape than Idaho's—the green land around the Mississippi River, a bit below St. Louis. Since the early 1900s, the Mississippi Lime Company of Ste. Genevieve, Missouri, has operated the biggest lime facilities in the country here: over one thousand acres of underground rooms eighty to one hundred feet deep. They produce more than a million tons of limestone a year, yet another rock source for Twinkies leavening that comes from ancient marine deposits. The limestone is removed by giant trucks, similar to the phosphate ore trucks in Idaho, that drive through immense, cavelike openings in the side of the limestone mountain. Calcium lime is one of the most essential chemicals in the world, used in the construction, steel, water treatment, chemical, pharmaceutical, paint, and paper industries as well as, of course, food. This is the calcium source for one of the leavening products that will be mixed in Chicago—the calcium in the monocalcium phosphate.

The newly mined limestone, calcium carbonate in its crude form (exactly what Tums® are made of), comes out in pieces as big as cars. It is crushed to football-size chunks in giant presses and carted in train cars up to the tops of nine tower ovens, some as much as eighty feet tall, encircled by catwalks and crisscrossed by long, angled conveyors.

Once dumped inside the kilns, the calcium rock is heated up to more than 2,000°F in order to drive off the CO_2 and transform the rock into calcium oxide (sometimes called lime, pebble quick-lime, or just plain quicklime). The newer ovens produce as much as ten tons an hour. That's a lot of lime. To get this kind of heat the full bottom third of some ovens is given over to pure flame. Fossil energy is a concern. After as little as two hours of baking, the resulting powdery "pebbles" of lime, now almost half their original mass, are crushed and screened for size. Rounded chunks one to two inches across are shipped off to places like the Chicago phosphate plant where they will meet up with the soda ash from Wyoming and the phosphoric acid from Idaho and Tennessee to be made into baking powder.

The pebble lime is loaded into sealed boxcars. It seems like overkill, enclosing mere rock like that, but precautions must be taken when you're dealing with quicklime, which is highly reactive. Left in the open, a pebble can turn into dust in a week's time. And there are other challenges inherent to quicklime: the lime companies learned a long time ago to keep the railcars absolutely dry. Apparently they first started shipping pebble lime in leaky, wooden freight cars. If it rained and the load got good and wet, the resulting chemical reaction generated enough heat to set the railcar on fire. New technologies always bring with them new challenges. Keeping your product from burning down the house, so to speak, is always a good place to start.

Ash for Twinkies

The third ingredient for Twinkies' baking powder, soda ash, comes to Chicago from FMC's Green River, Wyoming, trona mine and soda ash plant. After being conveyed about eight miles from the bottom of the trona mine previously described (both baking soda and soda ash come from trona), the ore is dropped onto piles the size of large houses at the Green River processing area. Bulldozers and front-loaders groan and roar as they push the piles into shape and back onto other conveyors up again and a half mile over to the soda ash plant. The conveyors look like sophisticated monorails, crossing fifty feet overhead, all bright white against the cobalt blue sky.

Boxy buildings house the mechanics for processing the trona, which is crushed, screened, boiled, clarified, filtered, dried, and cooked in a city-block-long, revolving tube of an oven; only then is it fine and pure enough (99.5 percent) to be called soda ash. As it cools down to different temperatures in a device called a crystallizer, it forms—what else?—crystals of different sizes, or eight grades, for hundreds of different end uses. They are colorless but reflect so much light that they appear bright white, like snowflakes. Today, it is one of the top ten inorganic chemicals produced in the United States, an essential ingredient in many industries including medical, oil-refining, and above all, glass-making. Sodium carbonate, aka soda ash, sal soda, or washing soda, has a long history of service to mankind.

For starters, prehistoric people were known to leach water through the ashes of burned plant stalks to obtain their primitive detergent for clothes washing, and the ancient Egyptians made glass ornaments with soda ash recovered from dried desert lakes. Green River soda use predates the mines: the Union Pacific Railroad tapped wells in the Green River, Wyoming, area for a crude, soda-based water softener for their steam engines in 1907. But glass-making has been its major use for centuries, and continues to this day. Soda ash, which is about 15 percent of the raw materials in glass, acts as a flux for the silica. About a quarter of the soda ash mined goes into container glass, and almost an equal amount into flat glass, fiberglass, and specialty glasses.

Still, another quarter of the soda ash processed goes into making other chemicals, often just to provide a base to balance off an acid, or as a reliable and not too expensive source of sodium. That is more or less what it does in Twinkies, where it is used to make chemical leavening. The other major use is, true to its ancient roots, for washing clothes—soda ash is also called washing soda, after all—and is a fundamental ingredient in many detergents as well as soaps and other cleaners, largely replacing the cruder and more expensive lye (the reason it is also used to digest wood pulp in the papermaking business). Interestingly, soda ash is also used to remove sulfur dioxide and hydrochloric acid from smokestacks by absorbing them in giant "scrubbers," which is ironic, considering that a few centuries ago, soda ash manufacturers generated these same pollutants. Specialized uses include sandblasting, hemodialysis filters, acid buffering in pharmaceuticals, and, of course, food products such as those in leavening.

This soda ash plant can produce more than 100 million tons of virtually pure sodium carbonate each year. Outside, a line of clean, white, sealed 100-ton hopper cars wait to be filled with fresh powder (FMC owns about 1,800 of them). Some of the hopper cars go to Kansas City to be made into sodium stearoyl lactylate, but the ones we care about right now are headed to Chicago to provide the sodium for sodium acid pyrophosphate, the third ingredient in baking powder.

The Salts Plant

On the industrial south side of Chicago, I am about to see how truckloads and trainloads of dangerous acid (phosphoric acid) and crushed rocks (lime and soda ash) become two similar, food-grade, bagged white powders, leavening agents ready to be baked into Twinkies or packaged into baking powder for the home cook:

sodium acid pyrophosphate (SAPP) and monocalcium phosphate (MCP). The fact that the manufacture of these two ingredients is so similar is not surprising. Both contain phosphate from phosphoric acid, and both are salts made by reacting a base with an acid—in this case, soda ash with phosphoric acid for the sodium acid pyrophosphate; lime with phosphoric acid for the calcium phosphate. The engineers refer to the place as a "salts" plant.

There's been a phosphate plant of some sort here since around 1900, but to say that there's been a tremendous change in techniques and raw ingredients over the years is to put it way too mildly. The original source of calcium was cow and pig bones (and perhaps teeth) from the nearby legendary Chicago stock-yards. The bones were boiled in sulfuric acid, which smelled awful and created toxic waste. But this plant is clean, odorless, modern and well-organized. Plain, low-cost apartment houses in need of maintenance and even a small, ramshackle farm sit nearby, bringing an odd, worn-down, urban/rural balance to the factory's industrial presence, what with its ten-story storage silos and chain-link fence gates.

Way in the back of the plant is a black, spherical tank filled with phosphoric acid: an acid-filled bowling ball the size of a house. The acid arrives in a constant chain of railroad tank cars lined up along the railroad siding, each holding more than 100 tons of the clear, oily, dangerous liquid. A massive array of pipes leads from this tank to the plant, a few hundred yards away. One set takes it to the part of the plant where the SAPP is made, another set to the MCP area.

Cyclone Activity

At a railroad offloading area on the far side of the plant, white soda ash hopper cars from Green River, Wyoming, are entering a covered area quietly, one at a time. Each railcar drops its load of sodium carbonate through a hole directly underneath it onto a basement conveyor, which dumps it into a five-thousand-gallon reacting kettle, along with a good dose of phosphoric acid. The resulting thick liquid, after passing through two different mixers, is cooked for an hour by spiraling through a thirty-foot-long, ten-foot-diameter, rotating oven that runs and rumbles twenty-four hours a day. The 450°F heat turns the liquid into crystals, simultaneously purifying it. A ceiling-high, funnel-shaped machine called a cyclone completes the drying and crystal-sorting process with a vigorous spin cycle.

The crystals are screened for various desired sizes, ranging from powder to saltlike. As with bicarb, crystal size is critical for each particular use. Of the dozen or so types, Donut Pyro® is one of the most interesting, invoking images of an overweight arsonist. Donut Pyro is what you need for making doughnut batter fluff up while being deep-fried. Though "pyro" normally implies something to do with fire, here it is a chemical term that means "chain of two," as in a single molecular chain formed from two separate phosphate molecules (phosphorus and oxygen) by the heat.

The plant is so automated that eerily, I see almost no one as we go dodging through a playground of augurs in stainless steel pipes. I finally spy a lone worker feeding empty bags to a robot that fills and stacks them on pallets, always remembering where it put the last bag and putting the next one neatly next to it, eight to a layer, ready for the bakeries. Dozens of similar products intended for industrial use fill a nearby warehouse, the route of one-third of baking powder.

Better Than Boiled Bones

Monocalcium phosphate, the other third of baking powder made here, starts at a second, covered rail dock, where hefty, sealed hopper cars full of loose, small, white-grayish, dusty rocks unload through their open bellies onto a subterranean conveyor belt. More rocks to eat. All the chunks are rounded and pock-marked. This is the limestone that has been processed into calcium oxide. The result is a nice, clean source of calcium, much more palatable than acid-boiled bones, and apparently much more efficient for baking powder than soybeans, sesame seeds, or milk. This mineral is so reactive that it seems almost alive. The pock-marks are the start of its reaction with the air. You can imagine it reacting with the acid.

With a low rumble, Innophos's conveyor whisks the pebble lime chunks into the basement, where they are pulverized, conveyed straight up, and then sent as a lumpy liquid via screw augurs in big pipes straight into the looming, five-thousand-gallon, stainless steel, enclosed kettles, along with phosphoric acid that has been piped in from the acid tank in back. The chemical reaction is instant and vigorous, as the lime and phosphoric acid are both obviously highly reactive. We're all wearing safety glasses and hard hats to protect ourselves from caustic or acid burns in case of an accident, and have removed all of our rings and watches not only as a security precaution but also because this is a food plant, despite its industrial feel, and there is zero tolerance for anything foreign that might tumble into the food containers.

Bucket and screw conveyors angle through the plant like so many flying attic rafters. But instead of being quiet as an attic, everything boinks and clanks and rumbles gently as the newly reacted chemicals are carried off to be dried in a room-size, rotating 250°F oven and packed into bags or "supersacks" (about a ton, filling out a big bag on a pallet) and shipped off to the cake-makers of the world.

Delicate powdered mixes made from phosphorus ore, sodium carbonate ore, and limestone, all dug from the ground, become an essential ingredient for baking light, fluffy cakes. It's a massive operation involving humming elevators, conveyors, ovens, and trains, all in the name of Twinkies, and not one bit of it suggests food. They could just as easily be making cement here, as far as an uninformed visitor is concerned. And why not, considering some of the ingredients?

Standing outside the plant gate, the point is clear: We eat rocks. Lots of rocks. And I'm about to go see another rock on the ingredient list, salt, brought up from deep underground without budging from the surface myself.

CHAPTER 17

Salt

There are three main ways to harvest salt, one of the several rocks we eat when we eat Twinkies. You can evaporate salt water to get crystals naturally—the oldest method—but that takes as much as two years of sunny, windy weather found only in limited (but beautiful) places. You can blast it out of a mine with dynamite and front-end loaders and then crush it, but that takes big mining operations and leaves a fairly impure rock salt suitable for water softening, ice control, and chemical processing—not food. Or you can flush it out of the ground with water and boil it down in an evaporation plant.

Only this last method, called solution mining, produces the fine, pure crystals of salt that we purchase at the grocery store or that are used in processed foods. Morton has a big facility devoted to this in the tiny, Victorian, one stop-sign town of Silver Springs, New York, near Rochester, that has been operating pretty much the same way since 1884. It is Morton's oldest facility, and it is one of the reasons that the Erie Canal, "the ditch that salt built" as they say, is nearby.

The table salt processed here is actually pumped out of the

ground as brine a few miles north, from various wells in the middle of a few fields, and sent by underground pipe to this facility. At this writing, the area is napped with a blanket of snow, providing a poignant contrast to Morton's solar salt facility in the Bahamas, one, which I readily admit, I'd prefer to visit this time of year.

Morton's plant is an agglomeration of nondescript industrial buildings, including a few that date from its Victorian days. The office building is gabled and brick (with a well-salted, ice-free walkway, of course) and some carved mahogany detail still surrounds a few of the older doors. The posts in a post-and-beam warehouse attached to the office look almost perforated with little slits. This is the former salt barrel–making loft, and for years, the barrel stave craftsmen tossed their axes into the posts as a quick way to hang them up. Pictures from 1911 featuring mustachioed and bowler-hatted workers line the current office walls, showing the perpetrators in action. This place reeks of history, and of course, salt has its own history—more ancient than Morton's.

A Dash Goes a Long Way

Salt is the most common and probably the oldest-known food additive. The first settlements of civilization were often made near salt outcroppings, licks that attracted animals and, as a result, our ancestors, who were interested in hunting said animals (hunters ate the salt their bodies needed by eating fresh meat). By 2000 B.C. our ancestors were salting meat, fish, and vegetables—including olives—to preserve them and to satisfy their healthy craving for salt. Salt played a major role in world trade among the ancient Greeks, Romans, and Chinese as much as 2,500 years ago, and in northern Europe since the 1300s, primarily for shipping fish. Wars were fought over it, and it was once as valuable as gold (early Chinese coins are said to have been made of it). Genoa and Venice rose to prominence as centers of the salt trade (and Silver Springs, too, in its own way). Through the centuries, the message has been clear: salt is not to be taken for granted.

While salt is also one of the basic tastes (salty, sweet, bitter, sour, and umami) and is necessary in our diet—our cells need it in order to function chemically—it is used as much if not more to simply enhance flavors, even sweet ones, like chocolate. That's why your chocolate fudge and cake recipes almost always call for a pinch of salt. In Twinkies, salt actually combines with sugar to make the cake and filling taste sweeter. But that's not all it does.

In Twinkies and in most home recipes for sponge cakes, salt is a functional ingredient, classified as a "processing aid," which means it enhances not only the flavor, but the texture as well. Salt helps bind the dough, helping provide uniform grain, texture, and strength, which allows the batter to hold more water and carbon dioxide and thus to expand more easily. Salt is not in Twinkies as a preservative, despite its historical pedigree for that.

Salt helps in as many as sixteen other essential food functions (one source at Morton says twenty-one), such as fighting bacteria and mold growth (a good bacteriostat, it is a traditional wound cleanser), activating and "setting" food coloring (think red hot dogs and hams; it is used extensively in textile dyeing, too), creating texture and rinds for cheese, acting as a binder for sausages, and, of course, as a preservative (think pickles and cabbage, as well as butter and fish). It works by absorbing moisture from bacteria and mold through osmosis, killing the cells or at least preventing them from reproducing. You add salt to bread dough to help control the yeast/sugar fermentation action (it acts as a chemical buffer or neutralizer) and to thus cut down on the big "voids," or bubbles. All of this is such a far cry from mere taste that it seems like salt doesn't get enough credit. Despite all of these chemical capabilities, salt is so benign that it is, in a way, the model for the large (seven hundred items) FDA class of food additives "generally recognized as safe" (GRAS), even though some argue that consuming too much of this household chemical can lead to increased blood pressure and heart disease.

The demand for salt is incessant: more than 200 million tons are mined annually worldwide. At more than 45 million tons per year, the United States is by far the world's biggest producer. Fewer than a dozen companies produce salt in the United States, and most are neighbors at the various underground salt deposits (born of ancient, dried-up seabeds) around the country.

Salt seems simple to us because it is common and familiar, but, in fact, these humble crystals are one of the most important industrial chemicals in the world and a key part of the modern industrial web. In 2003, according to salt industry experts, over two-thirds of the salt produced went to the chloralkali industry for transformation into other chemicals—notably chlorine via electrolysis, which is also used to bleach the cake flour in Twinkies (as described earlier) and to make the lye (sodium hydroxide) that is used to process a number of other Twinkie ingredients. Only about 5 to 6 percent of the salt produced is used for food products; 8 percent of evaporated salt goes to highway deicing, 12 percent to water conditioning, and 6 percent to agriculture. Its thousands of industrial applications include roles in making aspirin, plastic, paper, ink, leather shoes, dyes, shampoo, rubber tires, vinyl seat covers, catalytic mufflers, steel and aluminum manufacturing, gasoline processing, tile glaze, adhesives manufacturing, and on and on—the list is estimated at fourteen thousand specific applications. This range stems from the fact that most chemicals are used to make other chemicals, and salt is one of what scientists call the basic chemicals (along with petroleum, sulfuric acid, lime [from limestone], phosphates, nitrogen, and oxygen) that are used to make just about everything else, including other food ingredients.

What a twist of fate it is that such a common, chemically neutral and nutritionally important ingredient is made from a highly reactive chemical (sodium) and a corrosive, even poisonous chemical (chlorine). But that's what these inorganic salts are: the boring, stable, safe result of a marriage of materials that in their elemental states are often highly reactive, which is why they get together in the first place.

Table salt is one of the least processed food additives (the "processing" it undergoes is primarily to separate it from other rocks). Because salt is a mineral, it never goes stale and, contrary to popular belief, it doesn't taste any better or fresher if you grind it with a salt mill (though finer crystals dissolve faster, increasing the seasoning's intensity). Only sea salts that have not been purified, and thus are still bound with other minerals from seawater, taste different from regular table salt (fleur de sel has even more minerals than regular sea salt, hence its pronounced flavor). Salt is everywhere, it seems, in one form or another.

THE DEAD SEA OF NORTHERN NEW YORK STATE

Dan Border, Morton's facility manager, drives me a few miles through rolling, partially wooded terrain to show me where the salt comes from, which just happens to be prime upstate New York dairy farm country. Over the years, Morton bought the mineral rights to a few small dairy farms around their Silver Springs, New York, plant to provide access to the giant salt deposit underneath, putting in unobtrusive salt mining wells and pipelines without disrupting the local landscape. We thread our way through the groves of trees lining a snowy country road, and find ourselves at a fence gate that opens to well-maintained field lane.

Even though Morton owns it, a farmer still grows corn and hay there. Several brand-new blue sheds, placed a quarter mile apart, which shelter wellheads and pipeline valves, are all that interrupt the natural landscape. A group of connected wells is called a gallery, and the few along this pipeline feed brine back to the plant. Once the valves are in, engineers stop by routinely to check them. The fields themselves are left to the farmers and animals—cows and deer, mostly. There is a pretty pond off to the side and a lot of large, felled trees. It is evident that Morton is not the only builder on this plot of land: it shares the role with beavers, one of whom, not to be outdone by the guys from Morton, has built a beautiful and enormous lodge near a very sizable dam.

This particular salt deposit, a remnant of the layer that made the oceans salty, is 2,400 feet deep at this point (not quite half a mile), about 100 feet thick, and spread over about four states: New York, Pennsylvania, Ohio, and Michigan (and Ontario). Other major deposits are found around Texas, Oklahoma, Kansas, Louisiana, North Dakota, a few spots in the Southwest and California (Death Valley), and western Canada. (Almost all of Morton's pretzel salt comes from a mine in the aptly named town of Grand Saline, Texas.) However, the layer of salt is close to the surface only in some areas, and that's why upstate New York is one of the oldest and most successful American salt-producing areas. The purest part, "the salt zone," the stuff that the miners want, is only ten to fifteen feet thick.

We pull up to one of the new, trim, unpretentious blue sheds at the edge of the field and forest. Inside are two small Christmas trees of pipes and wheels and levers and gauges, much of which is wrapped in insulation. *This is it?* I think. The setup is so unassuming that except for the ten-inch pipe surrounded by concrete jutting out of the ground, it suggests a heating and cooling setup in a suburban garage rather than the high-tech mining operation that it is. Flowers of crystals abound on some of the simple plumbing at the wellhead, a mineral looking so much like ice it is hard to think of it as food.

A humble red plastic bucket, crusty from previous samplings, hangs from a small spout, offering a taste. Who wouldn't want to taste fresh salt as it comes out of the earth, direct from 2,400 feet below, on a winter afternoon, in the middle of a field? No pucker is as serious as the one produced by this water, dark gray with salt—and this pucker lasts—ten times as salty as seawater.

The art and the goal of the miner is to get as much salt into the brine and thus up the pipes as physically possible. That works out to about 2.6 pounds of salt per gallon of water—and this is at hundreds of gallons per minute. Too much salt and solids drop out. Too little, and it's inefficient to crystallize. It can take a few years of tuning the process to get the pressure just right and to find the purest salt in the deposit. As such, solution mining is fairly complex.

First, you drill two vertical wells into the salt deposit as much as a mile apart, and line them with steel and concrete to protect the local soil and groundwater. Then, you connect the two vertical wells with a horizontal bore, a feat of technical derring-do involving a torpedo-like, remote-controlled, steerable, self-powered, thirty-foot-long drill with rotating claws on its tip. The digger goes down the ten-inch pipe and takes a gentle turn in order to channel down into the middle of the salt deposit, reaching all the way over to the other vertical well. Imagine the challenge of sending this digging device down one pipe, through a few thousand feet of salt and then still managing to "hit" the second well—a minuscule, ten-inch-wide target a mile away. It must seem like directing a space probe to Mars, or at least like playing a very, very slow and expensive video game. (This same technology—directional drilling—enables the oil companies to dig under the tundra of the Arctic National Wildlife Refuge in Alaska from a reduced number of slightly remote platforms.)

Once the hole is drilled, water is pumped down the well (called an injection well) from the shed at a few hundred pounds of pressure. It dissolves and soaks up salt as it goes, working its way through the freshly drilled channel in the salt deposit. The stream of brine can be as much as two hundred feet wide near the injection wells, but narrows like a teardrop as it nears the second well; pressure forces the saturated brine to flow right up to the surface.

From that point, the brine flows along the pipeline a few miles back to the plant, where it is joined by other raw brine from the twenty-five or so other wells nearby. Other than a small gap in the trees here and there, which indicates where a pipeline lies underground, the gently rolling landscape is rural and undisturbed, peppered with prosperous dairy farms.

After all this effort, the brine ends up behind the plant, pouring rather unceremoniously from a big spigot into what looks like a large, shallow swimming pool. If you snuck a swim there you wouldn't need to worry much about sinking, it's so dense with salt: the Dead Sea of Silver Springs, New York.

CRYSTALS AND CARDBOARD

Here's where salt mining gets more complicated. Instead of being allowed to evaporate naturally under a hot summer sun, which is not very efficient in places like upstate New York, the brine feeds into a group of several five- to six-story-high, cone-bottomed, sixteen-foot-wide cylindrical vessels called evaporators, evaporator pans, or, more literally, forced circulation pans. These pans are cleverly designed to boil brine in a fancy heat exchanger made of a network of steam-heated titanium tubes. But "pan" is a misnomer—from the bottom they look like sixteen-foot-wide rocket ships encircled by gantries, or in this case, steel catwalks and staircases. I climb up five stories with salt engineer Dennis Grove—these things are *tall!*—on steel catwalks and steps (and down again and up again and around and down again and up again) to peer into a small porthole encased in thick glass at the top of this rocket ship. Though I am half expecting to see an astronaut's helmeted head and a gloved thumbs-up, I'm satisfied when only thick, dark gray-brown concentrated salt water splashes against the glass and drips slowly down. This, and what follows, is basically the same method developed here in 1884 by Joseph Duncan, Morton's predecessor, with only modest modern updates.

From there, condensed, white brine flows rapidly through a series of open tanks, giving new meaning to the term "white water." The impurities float off; the newly washed, dense salt crystals drop to the bottom and are piped out onto three rotating filter dryers in the noisiest room, where a 400°F blast zaps the last of the water from the salt mixture in half a minute. The salt looks kind of clumpy and heavy, not powdery, so it's not done yet. More blowers and more dryers await around the corner. At this point it can be conveyed by open belt conveyors or augurs (screw conveyors in pipes) to various processing points depending on the kind of salt being made. When little white piles of spilled salt accumulate beneath them, they are quickly swept up by workers.

Once dried, the slightly brown crystals form small cubes that reflect light so well they appear white. They are screened for consistent size on vibrating trays and then poured onto concave conveyors. Minuscule amounts of various additives may be mixed in—a mere dusting—as the salt passes through; things like potassium iodide (for iodized table salt) and/or an anticaking or free-flowing agent such as sodium silicoaluminate or calcium silicate, the stuff that keeps it pouring when it is raining, as the enduring Morton trademark says. Some salt is ground as fine as talcum powder for the bakeries, which demand the fast-acting quality.

In the older part of the plant, an upper loft floor is filled with solid cast-iron steel machines, many of which are painted a comforting forest green. Some are from the 1940s. With their gentle curves, they are much more pleasing to the eye than the brand-spanking-new, sleek but squared-off stainless steel ones nearby. This is the famous "round can department," where they make every part of the familiar blue cylinders found in grocery stores and kitchens—the cardboard tops, the little patented metal spouts, and so on—from scratch. Blank aluminum and cardboard coils are stacked on one side of the room, new containers on the other.

Downstairs, at the end of the production line, conveyors dump different varieties of salt (some with different-size crystals to meet customer specs; some with minuscule, trace amounts of additives such as iodine, dextrose to stabilize the iodine, or the anticaking agent sodium ferrocyanide, better known as yellow prussiate of soda) into hoppers that fill the fifty- or eighty-pound bags, or the two-thousand-pound supersacks, four-foot soft cubes on pallets, or load some directly into rail cars, or tank trucks—after a last trip through a metal detector—for shipment to the big bakeries and other food processors. The stream of salt pouring into a tank car is a foot wide.

Packing machines pull open the bags before a white whoosh fills them, almost instantly, and they are grabbed by robots that brusquely and hypnotically push and stack them on pallets. Then we dash off to the truck bays to watch forklifts load the pallets of bags and also cartons of the familiar blue canister into the waiting tractor-trailer trucks.

Sitting near a truck bay is an open, damaged carton; a blue can with the familiar little girl and her umbrella catches my eye. It is presented to me as a gift. It is still slightly warm. Its contents may very well have been underground this morning. Fresh salt.

But enough about simple, monolithic minerals that hardly need any processing. Now it's time to break up some fat.

CHAPTER 18

Mono and Diglycerides

Mono and diglycerides always appear as a pair on ingredient lists. What do they do, and why must they do it together? Why are they found in Triscuits®, peanut butter, and ice cream? And what role do they play in Twinkies? They are the old couple that turns up in thousands of processed foods.

OF MILK AND MOLECULES

Think of the best known, most basic, perfectly emulsified blends of fat and water: milk and its derivatives, butter and cheese. Mono and diglycerides are natural milk emulsifiers (the word "emulsion" is derived from the Latin word meaning "to milk out"). When great chefs like Gray Kunz (or you, of course) make a cream sauce, they include mono and diglycerides in their fancy, homemade sauce simply by using butter and cream.

While the name may be daunting, the words are easy to parse. Triglycerides (molecules made of one glycerin molecule and three fatty acids) are found in almost all fats, like butter and olive oil and soybean oil, but not all fats are triglycerides. The obvious example is mono and diglycerides, so named because instead of three fatty acids, the glycerin is attached to either one ("mono") or two ("di") fatty acids. They may be fats, but they are unusual fats, in that their job is to tie fat and water together.

Mono and diglycerides (M & D to us) are the most widely used synthetic emulsifiers in the world, having been perfected in the 1920s (lecithin, a natural emulsifier now refined out of soybean oil, comes in second). In baked goods, M & D create an abundance of small, uniform air cells for fine grain and softer, longer-lasting crumb, created in part by the reduction in surface tension between water and fat in the batter. They affect both the cooking and the dough's starches in ways that butter or oil alone cannot. They also work in minute percentages of a recipe—usually less than half a percent by weight—so they don't pose any dietary problems. These little things are *good*.

The list of other food applications for mono and diglycerides is impressive, although they are usually achieved while paired up with a similar product called sodium stearoyl lactylate (made in the same plant and described a little later on) and/or an emulsifier such as polysorbate 60—both of which are used in Twinkies, too. Various versions of mono and diglycerides can help improve batter stability (while waiting for oven time in an industrial bakery—they are the most powerful emulsifiers in bread), retard staling and extend shelf life (food companies' mantra), enhance the fat that's present so less fat is needed, reduce separation in icing, peanut butter, margarine and butter substitutes like I Can't Believe It's Not Butter!® or Lee Iacocca's Olivio®, stabilize fat in chocolate candy, and prevent clumping in artificial coffee creamer. Many ice creams, like Cold Stone Creamery's® and Edy's® Grand Light Rich & Creamy Vanilla incorporate M & D for extra smoothness (reducing the need for egg yolks and especially cream, the natural source of lush texture). Crisco needs them to aid in water solubility and to raise its melting point. They even work in plastic food containers like yogurt cups as an antistatic agent. No wonder they're on so many ingredient lists. And how nice that they are made from nothing more than vegetable oils.

Encountering Full Hydro

American Ingredients is one of the few specialized manufacturers of mono and diglycerides in the world. Its Grandview, Missouri, plant sits at the edge of the wide-open Kansas prairie, and, on the day I visit, a violent wind is blowing. As we stagger across the parking lot, Troy Boutté, Director of Research and Development, who holds a Ph.D. in food science, helps me get some basic and helpful facts down. "Mono and diglycerides are fats," he shouts. Simple enough. At the loading dock, my eyes are drawn to piles of what look like layers of puddled white wax around a big hose base, as if it were the base of a giant candlestick at the end of a long dinner. A big dipper ladle is nearby, also encrusted in white. I break some off, surprised to find that it is hard, more like plastic than wax, though a bit slippery. This is "full hydro," fully hydrogenated soybean oil, totally full of fat, which is why it is solid at room temperature. It's hard not to wonder if this is what the insides of your arteries would look like if you ate nothing but saturated fat.

It is not anatomy, though, that we are examining—only a loading dock in the windy Midwest prairie where big tank trucks hook up fat, braided, stainless steel hoses to their bellies and unload vegetable oils (mostly soybean—fully, partially, and nonhydrogenated) and also sunflower, palm, cottonseed, canola, or corn oil. There are two sets of pumps, hoses, and holding tanks for the oil—a separate set used to be reserved for kosher materials, but in the twenty-first century, most everything is kosher thanks to consumer demand, so that pump is out of service. American

Ingredients could use any fat to make mono and diglycerides, even a solid beef or pork fat like it used to, but to keep kosher it uses mostly soybean oil. For a manufacturer, and American is one of the major ones, all that matters is that the source is made of triglycerides. For a manufacturer, fat is fat.

From Soap to Cake

Glycerin is part of all fats, whether animal or vegetable. In 1783, the Swedish chemist Carl Wilhelm Scheele was the first to extract glycerin from a natural source, olive oil. Today, one of the biggest glycerin producers in the world is Procter & Gamble, which is no surprise because glycerin is a big by-product of soap-making, one of P & G's best-known businesses.

Soap is usually made from natural oil sources such as soybean as well as coconut, palm, palm kernel, canola, cottonseed, or olive oil, among others, including beef and pork fat. At one point in the soap-making process the fat is refined, or fractionated, which means the fat molecules are literally split up. It is an intriguing and surprisingly quick process that takes place in a three-foot-wide, eighty-foot-tall tower called a hydrolyzer. Superheated (500°F), superpressurized water is pumped into the top, while hot oil is pumped into the bottom. The reaction splits the fat into fatty acids and glycerin; the fatty acids are then drawn off the top and processed into soap or stearic acid (another Twinkie sub-ingredient), among other things, while the glycerin is pumped out the bottom for use as a food additive, but also in cosmetics (especially moisturizers), pharmaceuticals, and numerous industrial products. One of its more intriguing industrial uses is in nitro-glycerin; put a little of *that* into your cake and it will *really* rise. (Note: glycerin by itself is not explosive.)

Another intriguing coproduct (as Procter & Gamble likes to say) is making methyl esters (instead of fatty acids) when splitting off the glycerin. Methyl esters are used to make diesel fuel. Technically an alcohol, glycerin (also called glycerol, also spelled "glycerine," and obviously the root of the "-gylceride" suffix) is a clear, sweet, thick oil, like a heavy mineral oil or corn syrup, and is delivered to the mono and diglycerides plant by tank truck, pumped into tanks at the windy loading dock.

On its own, glycerin is a very useful food additive. Among other things, it works as a solvent for coloring, as a moistening agent for baked goods, and as a texturizer in syrup (its viscosity lends a desirable body). It prevents sugar from crystallizing in icings and candies, and, best of all, improves the texture and allows for the use of less sugar in lower-calorie ice cream.

Most of the glycerin used in the United States is made abroad in places as diverse as Mexico and Malaysia (from palm and palm kernel oil). Dow Chemical makes glycerin synthetically, from propylene gas, a petroleum product, at refineries in Freeport, Texas, and in Germany, but its process is, naturally, a trade secret. Food clients these days almost always want kosher glycerin, and yes, petroleum-sourced food is generally kosher. Why not? No matter which source, the pure glycerin is the same. And a bunch of it ends up in American Ingredients' Missouri plant, destined for greatness in cakes.

COOKING AND COOLING OIL

Reacting the oil and glycerin is pretty simple and quick. Once mixed at about a 3:1 ratio, the only requirements are high heat, an unnamed catalyst (reputed to be an alkali of some sort), and about half an hour in a two-story-high stainless steel tank. The plant is virtually automatic, somewhat dark, and filled with dozens of pipes going in and out of the various thirty-foot-tall stainless vats. Save for a couple of guys loading boxes at the end, almost no humans are on the floors and ladders. Meanwhile, the violent prairie winds play a symphony with the steel walls, giving life to an otherwise still scene.

In the next building, the hot, liquid M & D are cooled down and treated in various ways in order to create a variety of products with different forms, consistencies, and functions to suit bakeries' mixing needs. Powders are popular, but so are beads and "milk shakes" that turn into pastes or semisolids. And some are distilled in a vacuum molecular still, a five-story-high tank with three-foot-diameter vacuum pipes poking out of it. Boutté describes it in uncharacteristically vague terms as "kinda like making whiskey." The inspection porthole at the bottom is two feet across and securely shut with two dozen hefty and thoroughly intimidating bolts.

The most intriguing cooling method (reserved here for the distilled monoglycerides) uses the spray chiller, a round, room-size chamber with a conical roof fitted with what looks like a big vent fan and a conical bottom with a hole in the middle as well. It is not in use right now, so we climb up a few steep steel staircases to take a careful peek inside. Our voices echo ominously. With a smooth funnel of a bottom, it looks like something out of a *Star Wars* escape sequence. As the hot oil is atomized out of the opening at the top, it turns into solid, tiny beads as soon as it hits the cool air and is funneled right out the bottom.

The more common cooling method uses a flaker, a cool, rotating drum onto which the hot oil is sprayed and cooled to a solid within seconds. As the drum rotates against a blade on one side, kind of like a giant lathe, the sheet of wax is scraped off and crumbles into flakes that are conveyed to a nearby grinder and shaker that dumps it directly into a line of plastic bag/boxes on a snaking conveyor. Hydrated slightly to become a moist powder, it is perfectly suited to being mixed into cake batter; a sample of small, white granules cling to my fingertips, feel like sticky wax, taste like nothing, and leave a cloying aftertaste on the roof of the mouth, much like the feeling you get if you add too much artificial creamer to your coffee, or if you eat a whole spoonful of premade frosting from a can. All that emulsifying comes at a price.

The whole process, remarkably, takes less than two hours. This smooth, inseparable couple just glides on out to the bakeries, ready to mix. Most likely, they'll dance first along with one of their more intriguing partners, polysorbate 60.

CHAPTER 19

Polysorbate 60

When my daughter asked, "Where does polysorbate 60 come from?" I became, as you now know, determined to find out. Chemical-sounding and mysterious (what does the 60 stand for?), this ingredient was both a tease—and a challenge.

The two basic questions—where does it come from, and what does it do?—aren't easy to answer, partly due to modern business reality, partly due to complex science (it doesn't sound "chemical" for nothing). It's actually hard to suss out who makes it because so many large companies have merged, divested, then reacquired divisions, formed joint ventures, or outsourced manufacturing. Almost everyone I spoke with talked about background only, often because of impending or recent corporate musical chairs. One manufacturer's product information operator replied, in response to a request, "We're kind of in limbo as to who would handle product information right now." A technical support guy whose job description is to explain how PS 60 is manufactured ended an interview with the sketchy, CIA-like disclaimer, "I'm not sure if we even sell it any more." That's like Kraft neither confirming nor denying that it sells cheese.

Also intriguing was the discovery that, in such mergers, the actual manufacturing plants and personnel generally stay intact, while only the names on the buildings change. (One older plant I visited actually had two names at the gate and two sets of personnel who didn't acknowledge each other, even though the plant had no obvious boundaries or sectors. In a phone interview, each had professed ignorance of the other, and each had a different street address, so I was amazed to find them sharing a guardhouse and a barbed wire gate—and a plant site. Turns out that one company makes a subingredient, the other makes the final ingredient, and officially they are separate entities, like roommates who share a room and a fridge but not food.)

One company that will admit to making polysorbate 60 is currently referred to as Uniqema, located in an industrial park just under the Delaware Memorial Bridge, on Atlas Point, on the Delaware River, which turns out to be exactly where polysorbate 60 was invented.

Guns and Butter, or Praise the Filling and Pass the Ammunition

From the 1920s until the 1940s, mono and diglcyerides were the main emulsifiers favored by bakers. However, during World War II, glycerin, which is essential to M & D production, was in short supply, given how much was going into making nitro-gylcerin for ammunition. So, the country had to choose between bullets or babkas, and the bullets won. Emulsifier manufacturers needed to find a chemical replacement for glycerin.

During this time, the New Castle, Delaware–based Atlas Powder Company, an early corporate spinoff of the DuPont gunpowder and dynamite business (a trust that was broken up in

1912—one of the other spinoffs became Hercules, yet another Twinkies ingredient supplier [of cellulose gum]), was manufacturing explosives for blasting caps. Part of this process involved making mannitol, a sugar alcohol sweetener, through the electrolysis of sugar. Unfortunately for Atlas, this produced considerable by-product, which the company simply dumped into the Delaware River (much as cheese plants used to get rid of whey). But Atlas's scientists studied it and found it to be chemically close to glycerin. With just a little cooking it could replace glycerin as an emulsifier. But it did not emulsify all that well, and it was considered mostly an industrial product. It didn't stay on the back shelf for long, though.

The peaceful 1950s was a time of tremendous activity focused on finding more efficient food substitutes. Atlas modified its industrial emulsifier for food use, patented it, and polysorbate 60 was on its way as an additive. Though the plant has changed owners numerous times over the years, it still cranks out the good emulsifier, part of what is now about a 25-million-pound-a-year market for PS 60, and over 80 million pounds a year for all polysorbates.

GETTING CREAMY

We love smooth, creamy foods, particularly those full of fat, which coats the tongue and offers feelings of satisfaction and fullness. Butter, thick cream, and raw egg yolk are nature's emulsifiers; those magical ingredients that marry water and fat, moisture and grease, fill our cakes with creaminess and, as one rather poetic engineer at an emulsifier company put it, "put the whip in whipped cream." Polysorbate 60 does this, and more, replacing real cream and eggs (and their accompanying expense and perishability) in Twinkies' "creamy filling" and other products, such as Kraft Cool Whip®, Duncan Hines® Creamy Homestyle Cream Cheese Frosting, and Ken's® Steak House Creamy Italian Dressing with something equally magical—just not as, well, natural.

In many foods, polysorbate 60 works as part of a team with mono and diglycerides and sodium stearoyl lactylate (more to come on this ingredient later) to make what the pros call an emulsifying system. Each emulsifier is partnered in this system because each reacts differently to water or oil—sodium stearoyl lactylate loves water, while mono and diglycerides and lecithin love oil. Polysorbate 60 loves both, but is especially good at retaining water in something like creamy filling, where it surrounds a small water molecule with numerous smooth, creamy, luscious fat molecules and won't let go; it holds tiny air bubbles much the same way. It makes the filling stable as a rock.

And like most emulsifiers, PS 60 is so potent that it always ranks in the "2% or less" category on food labels, including Twinkies—it is regulated to less than 0.46 percent in most foods, 0.3 percent in salad dressings—meaning that it takes probably less than a hundredth of an ounce for PS 60 to work its magic in one little finger cake.

So, Where Does Polysorbate 60 Come From?

I'm relieved when I finally find a couple of engineers who can (and will!) identify exactly what it is they make and where they make it. As anticipated, polysorbate 60 is complex, but much to my surprise, also rather simple, as its basic ingredients come from corn, oil palms, and petroleum. It's the processing, as you might expect, that one of the technical specialists says, is "a little more complicated than your average chemistry."

Corn Again

Sorbitol—a popular, pleasant-tasting, reduced-calorie bulk sweetener that does not cause tooth decay—comes from corn, or rather, dense dextrose corn syrup like that which is made in the wet milling plants in the Midwest. Check your chewing gum, cough syrup, and toothpaste ingredient labels and you'll likely find it. Technically a sugar alcohol (which is why it doesn't do a number on your teeth), it's a popular ingredient in pharmaceuticals and cosmetics, too—as a humectant, to keep moisturizers moist, or as a thickener, for shampoo or conditioner.

Sorbitol is not harvested, though a French chemist apparently discovered it in mountain ash berries back in 1872, a few years after sorbic acid, another Twinkie ingredient, was also found in those berries. The largest manufacturers are specialists like SPI Polyols, which since the 1990s has shared facilities with the Uniqema polysorbate plant on Atlas Point in New Castle, Delaware. All SPI really does to the corn syrup is hydrogenate it, just as soybean oil is hydrogenated to make shortening, only at much higher temperatures and pressures. Then it pumps it over to Uniqema.

But the corn syrup is only hydrogenated minimally, as a couple of hydrogen atoms are forced onto each molecule. The whole process takes no more than a couple of hours, and doesn't smell or make noise, although when it's discharged, the corn syrup does smell sweet, for a perfectly logical reason. "It smells like you're cooking sugar syrup, because that's what you're doing," says Mary Lou Cunningham, a chemical engineer at SPI Polyols.

Separation Anxiety

If stearic acid, the second ingredient found in PS 60, were the only ingredient, you *could* say PS 60 grows on trees—trees on

Malaysian oil palm plantations, planted in orderly rows by the thousands. Most stearic acid is made from the oil derived from the palm tree, but any vegetable oil works, as does tallow (it's the triglyceride that does the trick). The name "stearic" is, in fact, derived from the Greek word for tallow.

Kuala Lumpur Kepong Berhad, or KLK, is one of the largest suppliers of palm oil (palm oil is derived from the "meat" of the oil palm fruit while palm kernel oil, which is produced at less than a tenth the volume of palm oil, is pressed from the seed). Like so many palm oil outfits, KLK started as a rubber company, incorporated in England back in 1906. In a wildly unusual effort at diversity, it now also owns Crabtree & Evelyn, the British manufacturer of skin care and gift food items that range from toiletries to tea—as well as over 370,000 acres of plantation, most of which was formerly rubber plantations and some of which was formerly natural rain forest. In general, about half the world's palm oil comes from Malaysia and much of the rest from Indonesia.

Oil palm fruit is plum-size and grows in reddish-orange bunches the size of basketballs that clump at the top of the palm tree's stump and at the base of the spreading fronds. Oil palm bunches can weigh more than 100 pounds, and the trees often stand over sixty feet tall. Workers wielding long bamboo poles with sickles attached to each end slice the bunches off, allowing them to fall for collection.

In Malaysia, the fruits then pass through a machine called a digester, after which the resultant mush is crushed in order to get the palm oil. Then, the oil is dehydrated, cleaned, and refined, and shipped overseas to a stearic acid or soap-making factory, such as the Twin Rivers Technologies plant in Quincy, Massachusetts, just south of Boston. Since palm oil is already about 49 percent saturated (palm kernel oil is 81 percent saturated), it doesn't require hydrogenation; it is naturally thick and stable, which is why it's long been a popular ingredient in margarine, shortening, and candies, especially in Europe.

To make stearic acid, it undergoes a refining process most commonly used to make soap. "It's really pretty simple," engineer Dave Astraukas tells me as we drive around the Quincy plant. (Apparently, slicing and dicing molecules in a complex refinery is child's play to him.) High heat plays such an important role—and it is already close to 100°F the day I visit—that we stay inside his air-conditioned Jeep as we tour the refinery.

First, the oil is broken down, or hydrolyzed, with superhot water (500°F) in an eighty-foot tower called, naturally, a hydrolyzer. The reaction is swift. The glycerin is drawn off and most of it sent to be made into soap but also into mono and diglycerides or pure glycerin. The fatty acids are separated in an even bigger, staircase-enrobed tower known as the fractional distillation tower, just as refined oil is separated into "fractions" like aviation fuel and gasoline in petroleum refineries. Stearic acid is one of those fractions, pumped hot around the corner to become fully hydrogenated, just like soybean oil is for shortening.

Because the stearic acid is now full of hydrogen, it is pumped as a hot liquid into waiting trucks that rush off to make quick, nearby deliveries before it cools (the rest goes into waiting railcars for shipment cross-country). The stearic acid will cool into a waxy solid on those trips, and will have to be melted by pumping steam into the walls of the railcars for half a day so that it can reliquefy. Besides the role it plays in PS 60 and other emulsifiers, stearic acid provides hallmark gooeyness for many shampoos and lotions, like Dove® Beautifully Clean Shampoo and Neutrogena® Norwegian Formula® Hand Cream. But at no point do I glimpse any oil, nor, for that matter, any hint of food. All I see are pipes, towers, and railcars—modern industry at its finest.

Mother of Polysorbate 60

Now that the corn syrup and the palm oil have been hydrogenated, pressed, hydrolyzed, fractionated, and hydrogenated again, they are ready for mixing. At the polysorbate plant, such as Uniqema's in New Castle, Delaware, corn syrup and palm oil are pumped at a temperature of almost 500°F into six-thousand-gallon reactor vessels and blended with a secret, proprietary catalyst for ten hours. What emerges are tens of thousands of pounds of thick, waxy liquid sorbitan monostearate, or SMS. (The name includes "mono" because only one "mole," a measure of weight, is attached to the sorbitol molecule; sorbitan tristearate, for example, has three moles. Moles are used for measurement because it is apparently easier to weigh a bunch of atoms than it is to count them.)

SMS, a weak emulsifier also known as sorbitan ester or sorbitan fatty acid esters, is the glycerin replacement that Atlas discovered years earlier. You can still find it in bread, icing, whipped toppings, ice cream, and cake mixes, as well as in plastic lubricants, usually paired with polysorbate 60 because of its mildness. When chemists learned that the petrochemical ethylene oxide reacted with other chemicals to make them water soluble, they tried it on SMS, and polysorbate 60 was born. That's what's now in store for the SMS at this plant. But securing ethylene oxide isn't necessarily so simple.

Domestic Oil

Twinkies share a subingredient with the most common plastic, made from the most used petrochemical in the world, and that's saying a lot. The oil companies mainly use natural gas as a source of ethane, a basic gas element, but also oil, depending on pricing and availability. Ethane is transformed almost instantly into ethylene. When the ethane arrives at the ethylene plant, which is generally located right by the refinery, it enters a steam cracker and is heated up to almost 1,400°F for only a millisecond in order to be transformed. That's quick. (An alternative source is ripening fruits like apples and bananas, but your fridge can't compete with ExxonMobil.)

Dow Chemical, the second largest chemical company in the world, Equistar, and others buy ethylene, or sometimes ethane or even the oil itself, from the oil refineries to make more than 11 million tons of ethylene oxide each year, at plants whose locations they would not identify for security reasons. Ethylene oxide is an excellent but entirely unlikely food chemical, seeing as it is highly explosive (it was used in tunnel-busting shells during the Vietnam War), a known human carcinogen, and a respiratory, skin, and eye irritant.

Ethylene and oxygen are mixed—carefully—in a forty-foot-long cylindrical reactor filled with a catalyst, a thin layer of silver on an alumina, silica, or ceramic base in the shape of thousands of ⅜-inch-diameter pellets, packed into inch-wide tubes within the reactor. The EO is then cooled and liquefied so some can be shipped in special, protective cylinders to the polysorbate plants, but the bulk of it is used to make polyester fibers and PET, the plastic in our ubiquitous soft drink and water bottles. Much of the rest goes into ethylene glycol for antifreeze, polyurethane foam, and brake fluid. Though food use is a relatively minor part of the picture, without ethylene oxide we simply would not have our favorite creamy filling. It's essential for turning a ho-hum emulsifier into a veritable powerhouse.

Pressure Cooking

In an undisclosed location, perhaps in an industrial park near Chicago, maybe in rural, central Pennsylvania, possibly in riparian Delaware, in a plant full of tanks, railroad sidings, and a maze of pipes and catwalks, big, stainless steel vats are filled with fresh, hot, luscious, liquefied sorbitan monostearate. Along with the pressurized and liquefied ethylene oxide, it is carefully pumped under high heat and pressure into closed, cylindrical, stainless steel reaction vessels called autoclaves. These high-tech tanks, which can range in size from one thousand to four thousand gallons and stand up to forty feet tall, are designed not only to handle heat and pressure, but to control any possible explosive tendencies expressed by the ever-ready-to-react ethylene oxide. All air is excluded by creating a vacuum in the vessel first. When I remark to a laconic chemical engineer at one of the manufacturers that this seems particularly dangerous, he says, "So are most other chemical reactions." Still, this is probably the most dangerous of the reactions that contribute directly to the Twinkie ingredient list.

After some deodorizing and purification, out pours a greasy, tan goo: polysorbate 60, ready to be mixed with oil and water. I'm warned not to taste a sample. It is so bitter, and the aftertaste on the back of your tongue so cloying, that an engineer sternly cautions me, saying "You won't be able to taste your dinner for a week." Could polysorbate 60 in the filling be the reason why Twinkies' taste seems to linger long after you've eaten one?

Parsing the Name

With the manufacturing figured out, it is finally possible to understand where this ingredient's intimidating name comes from: "poly" means it is a polymer, or something with a long, and in this case, synthetic, molecule; "sorb" obviously comes from "sorbitol"; "ate" means that oxygen is now tacked on to the molecule; and "60" differentiates this product from polysorbate 20 or polysorbate 80, which, being made from different vegetable oils, are each cooked up a bit differently and are suited for different uses. PS 80 and PS 20 boast similar attributes—PS 80 smooths out cake mixes, icing, such as Betty Crocker® Whipped Vanilla Frosting, and ice cream, like Eskimo Pie® Ice Cream Bars, which are lacking in eggs and cream; PS 20 emulsifies soaps, shampoos, and skin care products like Neutrogena® Oil-Free Acne Wash, but primarily due to its soapy taste is not a food additive. Almost all PS 60 is used in food, but some can be found in lotions like Jean Naté® Hydrating Body Lotion or Olay® Moisturinse™ Shower Body Lotion.

Surprisingly, even most chemical engineers don't know where the numbers 20, 60, and 80 come from, including the head of technical services for one of the world's largest polysorbate manufacturers, who shall remain unidentified out of courtesy. Some digging shows that it is pretty simple after all. The first digit, or the "ten" in each name—2, 6, and 8—is the "one" digit in the number of carbon atoms in each source's oil molecules: coconut oil, which is made into lauric acid, has 12 carbon atoms and is used to make polysorbate 20; olive oil, which yields oleic acid, has 18, and is used to make polysorbate 80. But here's the glitch, or so it seems: soybean and canola oils, the most common oils in Twinkies' polysorbate 60, have 18 carbon atoms. The aforementioned head of technical services finds this equally vexing, until we realize that the *original* recipe for polysorbate 60 called for beef or pig fat (tallow or lard), which contain 16 carbon atoms (therefore, polysorbate 60).

And there we have it: polysorbate 60—or polyoxyethylene (20) sorbitan monostearate—explained and demystified. Seems it *does* grow on trees, after all. I can't wait to tell my kids. That'll be easy. What I'll have a harder time explaining is where artificial vanilla and butter come from.

CHAPTER 20

Natural and Artificial Flavors

In order to make flavors, you need raw materials from places as diverse as tropical islands and Chinese or Gulf Coast oil fields. In order to appreciate flavors you need a nose, a tongue, and a brain. In order to fully *understand* flavors, you need a degree in chemistry and access to some sophisticated electronic testing equipment.

Tasting Twinkies is complex. Only our senses of smell and taste can detect chemicals—the others (sight, sound, touch) rely on physical impact—so it makes sense that all flavors, even those that are naturally occurring, are chemical. In fact, Joyce Kiley, a flavorist who runs Flavor Sciences Inc., a flavor supplier in Stamford, Connecticut, confirms what anyone who's ever had a cold has experienced firsthand. "You taste with your nose," she says, which can not only detect thousands of different odors but is "99 percent accurate" (although Kiley confesses to supporting her nasal talent with the use of a gas chromatograph that analyzes the molecular makeup of an odor, an option unavailable to most consumers). This observation dovetails somewhat with color experts' adage that "we eat with our eyes first." The importance of the eyes and nose in the gustatory experience makes you question how necessary the tongue actually is, given that the tongue can only handle the five basics—sweet, sour, bitter, salty, and umami, or savory—while the more sophisticated olfactory sense goes much further, elevating mere taste to flavor.

Memory is also important to taste and, certainly, satisfaction. When we eat a favorite snack cake, we expect it to taste exactly as we remember it from last time, or from childhood. Marketers of processed foods like Twinkies know this well, and take it to heart. The look, the flavor, the texture of a snack cake must be consistent, even over decades. And if consumers want it to taste "like homemade," in Twinkies' case, it better taste buttery. For a buttery taste without real butter and its attendant spoilage and expense, manufacturers use (surprise!) artificial flavors. For a slightly richer or deeper taste, bakers add a dash of natural flavor, as is no doubt done with Twinkies' vanilla, hence the ingredient listing of "natural and artificial flavors." Hedging your bets is good business.

Figuring out how to achieve the desired taste, from apple to walnut, in products that entail extreme cost control, automated mixing, extended holding, fast baking, and long shelf life, all of which can destroy flavors, is no small feat. For this, the big bakeries turn to flavorists,[11] or flavor chemists, like Kiley at Flavor Sciences, Nancy McDonald of M&M Consulting and Laboratory of Apopka, Florida, or staffers on the payroll of the many major flavor companies, such as Sensient Technologies, in Indianapolis, Indiana, or McCormick and Company of Sparks, Maryland.

---

11. Several of the professionals I spoke with willingly tasted Twinkies, often for the first time since they were kids, and though they usually scoffed at their own diminished desire for such sweet things, they were impressed with Twinkies' successful blend of flavors. One renowned flavorist, consultant to the biggest consumer food product companies in the world (who shall remain anonymous for obvious reasons) offered the following (technically and scientifically accurate) assessment upon a Twinkie tasting: "Gee, that's *great!*"

The flavorists I challenged, including Kiley and McDonald, all agree that Twinkies incorporate only two flavors, vanilla and butter, with butter existing primarily in the cake part and vanilla primarily in the filling (as noted in the Note to the Reader, Hostess will neither confirm nor deny). Any other flavors, they deduced, would result from baking. Flavorists rely on their senses to make this kind of statement, and they can make it right after just one taste. If I paid them a lot of money (not likely), the flavor profile and constituents could be analyzed on a gas chromatograph and/or a mass spectrometer and graphed out precisely, which is what consultants and flavor companies do all the time.

Incidentally, according to Hostess, vanilla wasn't even the principal flavor of the original 1930 Twinkies filling—for the first ten years, banana was. But World War II created such an extreme shortage of bananas that the song "Yes, We Have No Bananas" soared to the top of the charts, and Hostess switched to the more widely available vanilla flavoring. So vanilla—both natural and artificial—and artificial butter are the agreed-upon flavors to investigate.

Thanks to a strong combination of homeland security (mostly inspired by the Bioterrorism Act of 2002—flavors are very concentrated, and thus one of the first things to safeguard) and fierce competitiveness in an arcane, artful science, plant and lab visits are simply out of the question. Not one flavor company would open its doors to me, and some won't even speak via phone to outsiders. My top contenders—flavor giants Rhodia, McCormick, and International Flavors and Fragrances (IFF)—explicitly declined any participation in research for this book. Luckily, a good number of professionals were eager to talk, on background, about their life's work. And what they do smells simply terrific, even if how they do it is terrifically complex. Even when it's all natural.

216 CHEMICALS AND IT'S STILL NATURAL

Flavors are pure chemistry. What you smell when you walk into a shop such as Bath & Body Works that sells candles, soaps, and incense are alcohols, aldehydes, acids, ketones, esters, phenols, furans, lactones, and assorted other hydrocarbons with names unfamiliar to most of us. And those are just *groups* of chemicals, not individual chemicals. They are also exactly what you smell when you sniff a Twinkie prior to devouring it. When you smell ripe or rotten fruit, you are smelling ethyl acetate, which is an ester and, depending on which kind you're talking about, either grows on trees or is made in oil refineries from natural gas. Alone, it is flammable and moderately toxic; mixed with other chemicals, it is rendered safe and smells like fruit. All of these chemicals are both natural and synthetic, and there's no escaping the terminology.

The main and most important ingredient in both, vanillin, is the same chemically, but the natural flavor has hundreds of other components as well, perhaps over 250; so many, in fact, that it is not completely understood (vanilla is not unique in this—coffee has more than eight hundred and is no better understood).

At the Rutgers University Center for Advanced Food Technology in New Jersey, scientists using a powerful gas chromatograph and flame ionization detector (and perhaps a Captain Cosmo Decoder Ring) positively identified 216 of natural vanilla's flavor components, including (of course) more vanillin than anything else, but also an astoundingly complex chemical list that includes literally dozens of organic compounds—maltol, catechol, ethyl vanillin, phenol, heliotropin, diacetyl—all of which are reassuringly part of the artificial vanilla recipe. One study classified, among others, 25 alcohols, 11 aldehydes, 20 acids, 10 ketones, 5 esters, 10 phenols, 10 furans, 2 lactones, and 40 miscellaneous hydrocarbons, including the basic aromatic compounds of natural gas, all found naturally in a lovely tropical orchid, not some contrived industrial product.

Each chemical contributes to what the pros call its bouquet—what we actually smell—even in the most minute of trace amounts. Some touches are so small that they barely register on the most sophisticated of equipment, not to mention in our noses. Only a minority surpass concentrations of 1 part per million. But when they are all mixed together, they help each other to smell and taste uniquely alluring.

Natural vanilla is probably the world's most labor-intensive agricultural product, and its plant-to-factory route is rather tortuous, considering it's a naturally occurring substance. Vanilla beans, which are actually not beans at all but the fruit of the only tropical orchid in the world to bear fruit—are famously difficult to grow and process. Vanilla only grows in tropical, equatorial climates, where the flowers are pollinated by hand in hillside gardens, a technique discovered in 1841 in French Madagascar. The delicate act takes place between dawn and noon on the *one* day in its life that the flower opens (the unlucky flowers drop to the ground). The beans first ripen on the vine for nine months before being harvested green and flavorless, when the curing process begins. They are dried for three to six months in special boxes and the open air, and are brought in each night and when it rains. Each pod is turned by hand as needed. Curing is an art but technically a way of inducing natural enzymatic action, or fermentation, to create aroma. The whole process can take five to six years from planting to sale. And this takes place mainly on the other side of the world from Twinkies' U.S. factories, in Madagascar, which supplies a whopping 60 percent of the world market (Indonesia supplies 30 percent). The rest comes from places like Tahiti, not much closer to Twinkies' bakeries, either.

Unsurprisingly, prices are in the hundreds of dollars per pound and are dramatically affected by Madagascar's weather, both meteorological and political (prices went up 500 percent after a recent typhoon reduced the crop by 40 percent). Vanilla is not only a difficult plant to grow and process, it is a difficult business, too. Only about two thousand tons are produced yearly around the world, and that varies with natural disasters and recipe changes in soft drinks (the 1985 introduction of New Coke, which eschewed the natural stuff, nearly broke the Madagascar economy with the attendant drop in demand). It is expensive enough that most food companies avoid using it wherever possible, but they, like Hostess, end up needing a tiny bit of it for an extra depth of taste that the artificial stuff can't seem to provide.

Vanilla is by far the single most popular flavor in the world, and the United States is by far its principal consumer. (Introduced to the United States via France, it was Thomas Jefferson who brought some back with him in 1789 after his gig as ambassador ended.) Once harvested, the beans don't go right to the bakeries. The natural vanilla used by the big food companies, as in most home recipes, is vanilla extract in liquid form. In contrast to the growing and curing of the beans, making vanilla extract is simple. The beans are chopped up into half-inch square bits, soaked in alcohol (ethyl alcohol, fermented from corn syrup) that percolates through it for about forty-eight hours, if heat is used, and weeks, if using a cold process. Matt Nielsen, head of Nielsen-Massey Vanillas, a family-owned, artisanal producer with fewer than fifty employees, uses the cold process in a room full of ten-foot-high stainless steel vats in Waukegan, Illinois, in order to make a few hundred gallons of high-quality extract at a time. McCormick, with 8,500 employees, the world's largest publicly owned flavor company, and other major producers or suppliers to companies like Geneva, Switzerland–based Firmenich Inc., the world's largest private flavor and fragrance company, with 4,760 employees and fifty locations, are more likely to use heat, along with more and bigger vats. (When asked if the neighbors complain about the smell, the companies claim they love it.)

Vanilla extract is precisely defined. The FDA requires a minimum of 13.35 ounces of vanilla beans per gallon, made up with a minimum of 35 percent alcohol (and 65 percent water). Some of the better beans are extracted with more alcohol to bring out the flavor, and some brands add sugar or corn syrup to take the edge off the alcohol or to act as a stabilizer. The alcohol, which is bitter to taste, evaporates during baking. Contrary to what some enthusiastic vanilla ice cream lovers may wish to believe, Nielsen confirms that the tiny bits of vanilla bean in some high-end brands of ice cream are there for impression only—they are *not* the flavorful seeds that we might think they are, but ground-up pods that were used to make the extract that actually flavors the ice cream.

OIL REFINERIES, NOT ORCHID GROVES

The name 4-hydroxy-3-methoxybenzaldehyde is not very elegant for the synthetic equivalent to the fruit of a beautiful tropical orchid. This is vanillin, and rather than hailing from exotic islands, just about all of it is made in two major petrochemical plants in China and one in Baton Rouge, Louisiana (the only place it is made in the United States). And most of *that* is made by one company, Rhodia, a French-owned, $6 billion-a-year, global chemical company with more than twenty thousand employees. (Rhodia owns the Louisiana plant and just in 2005 bought one of the two Chinese plants, in Zhejiang province, just west of Shanghai.) Besides being the backbone of the most popular ice cream flavor, vanillin is the most common aroma chemical in the world. For well over a hundred years, we haven't been able to live without it.

Vanillin was first synthesized in 1875, only about twenty years after it was first isolated and identified in the natural world. Originally, vanillin was painstakingly cooked (in Germany) from coniferin, those sugary crystals on pinecones that give off a slight vanilla smell. In the 1890s, a French chemist (not a chef, mind you) found a way to make vanillin from clove oil. (If you *really* smell it you can see how they are related.) For years vanillin was extracted in the form of lignin from wood as a by-product of papermaking, but now less than 10 percent, and maybe only 5 percent, of food-grade lignin comes from wood pulp these days. It is actually cleaner and easier to make it from hydrocarbons (petroleum) because of all the sulfuric acid and energy needed to process pulp.

As noted, most flavor companies won't talk, but fortunately, some are more accommodating, including Firmenich, the third largest of the flavor companies (founded in 1895). Mike Cadwell, senior flavorist in its Anaheim, California, office, is glad to help explain how these flavors are made.

Chemically, vanillin is an oxidized alcohol, a (luckily distant) cousin of formaldehyde. Economically, its popularity is a no-brainer: it costs about one-two-hundredth of its natural counterpart because it is about two hundred times as strong, depending on what strength natural vanilla you compare it to (less than an ounce to a gallon is a common but inaccurate measure). Aesthetically, most food scientists agree, the artificial version never quite develops the full flavor of its natural counterpart, though it does survive the high heat of baking better than the natural version does. But since Madagascar became to vanilla what Saudi Arabia is to oil some time around the 1960s, the price difference is too profound for the big food companies to ignore, and the use of artificial vanilla flavoring has since taken off.

Artificial vanilla manufacturing starts a long way from the flower fields, with crude oil and one of its basic components, benzene, a colorless, sweet-smelling, flammable liquid solvent, one of the so-called aromatic compounds found in flowers, fruits, and vegetables as well as in crude oil (the major source), natural gas, and coal tar. Cadwell says of these delicate scents, "Most are straight from the dinosaurs." Benzene is the source of feedstocks for thousands of products including vanilla flavoring, artificial colors, gasoline, and that symbol of clean chemistry, aspirin. But as straightforward as this may sound, it's important to note that making benzene is a bit dangerous: not only is it a known carcinogen, but in March 2005, a benzene tank at a refinery in Texas City, Texas, exploded, killing fifteen and injuring 170.

Whether in Baton Rouge or just west of Zhejiang, making vanillin is complex and not at all appetizing. In fact, it is almost impossible to view as a food process. At the refinery, benzene is oxidized at the steam cracker and reacted with propylene (also from petroleum) to get cumene, an important industrial chemical, which is then further reacted to get phenol, a clear, sweetish-tarry-smelling liquid that used to be sold under its common name, carbolic acid, as a sore throat remedy (it was the first surgical antiseptic used by Sir Joseph Lister, who invented the mouthwash that still bears his name). Phenol is still used in antiseptic products; it was reacted with formaldehyde to make the first plastic, Bakelite, too, but is now mostly used to make polycarbonates (including CDs) and plywood glue, with leftovers going into artificial vanilla.

The chemical reactions in the name of food continue in the same refinery-like plant. The phenol is condensed into white crystals called catechol, an oily methyl ester used in photographic developers, which is liquefied and catalyzed into guaiacol, a yellowish semisolid, light-sensitive alcohol that has a slight smoky/woody/spicy vanilla scent. This is dried into off-white crystals or liquefied and sold by the major chemical companies to the major flavor companies for further processing into vanillin. Guaiacol is a popular chemical with the pharmaceutical companies, too, who make it into guaifenesin, which you might recognize as a popular decongestant used in the cough and cold elixirs that line the shelves in your local drugstore. It might work for cough syrup, but not for Twinkies, not yet.

Next, the guaiacol is reacted under high temperature and pressure with a dash of the corrosive, solid glyoxylic acid so a sweet cherry hint (or "note") develops in addition to the almost delicate, sweet benzene odor. And bingo: bright, white, aromatic vanilla-smelling crystals drop out of the liquid. Pure vanillin, if you can call something synthetic pure.

A scientist at one of the big firms who insisted upon anonymity explains this oil-refining/chemical process in almost artisanal terms: "You go from medicinal to woody notes to sweet woody notes to smoky sweet and then vanilla, which is a combination of all these things. It's a nice progression." Except that instead of mixing little test tubes in a lab or aging wine in oak barrels, this is done in giant, off-limits chemical plants with towers and tanks and railcars coming and going—not to mention the ever-present risk of detonation.

Building a Flavor

The pure artificial vanillin can't quite fully substitute for natural vanilla, not yet. First, it must be mixed or cut with other flavors to become more palatable and to more closely resemble real vanilla, with its hundreds of subtle components. Evidence of this can be found on the labels of imitation vanilla sold in grocery stores: every producer blends it a bit differently to please each of its big customers in terms of price, performance, and aroma.

My favorite ingredient on the label of bottles of artificial flavor such as vanilla is the seemingly redundant term "artificial flavor." This begs a philosophical (or perhaps grammatical) question, implying that if the second artificial flavor was *not* added to the first artificial flavor, then perhaps the first artificial flavor might not be artificial, or might not even exist.

In an example of chemical incestuousness, what's added tends to be some of the very same intermediate or precursor chemicals used to make vanillin in the first place, put back in to round it out: guaiacol; ethyl maltol, a powdered, white sweetener that smells like caramel, jam, strawberries, and burnt toast (some say cotton candy) made from an oily, aromatic chemical with the energy-packed name furfural, which is itself distilled from oat hulls, corncobs, sugarcane stalks, or wood that has been treated with sulfuric acid; or heliotropine, another white, crystalline refinery product similar to vanillin, an aldehyde with a cherry and floral scent that suggests heliotropes, a popular kind of garden plant, as well as the distinctive smell of Tahitian vanilla (it is also popular in perfumery). These flavor chemists go deep not into tropical jungles but into organic chemistry to make their products sing.

Artificial vanilla also needs to be mixed with some additive to smooth it out, thicken it, and keep it moist. McCormick® Pure Vanilla Extract, along with supermarket brands like Stop & Shop's, uses corn syrup. Some add caramel color. Many other brands use the decidedly unfoodlike-sounding additive propylene glycol (also found in artificial colors). Colorless, odorless, and oily, it's a great additive, a solvent (an alcohol based on glycerin) that is so safe it's used in cosmetics and medicines as a moisturizer, as well as in personal or sexual lubricants. It's also the primary ingredient in the "paint" inside a paintball and the fuel for theatrical smoke machines, among other industrial applications (not to be confused with its sister, ethylene glycol, the main ingredient in automobile antifreeze). And it comes from a rather industrial source: oil refineries.

Propylene glycol, a kind of alcohol called a diol, is made by Equistar and Dow Chemical, the biggest producer in the world (worldwide annual capacity: more than a billion pounds), in half a dozen Gulf Coast petrochemical plants in Texas and Louisiana. Like most everything else in this flavor, it is made from petroleum at a refinery in a violent and unfoodlike process that varies from place to place and time to time. One common way is to "crack" natural gas under a flash of high heat and crack it again to separate out propylene gas, which is then reacted with chlorine and lye (or sometimes hydrochloric acid—all are chemicals made from salt, another useful Twinkie ingredient) to become a liquid, propylene oxide. The PO is then reacted with that old chemical standby, water, to make propylene glycol.

But vanilla is only half of the flavor added to Twinkies. It takes butter to complete the taste, no matter that there is no real butter in a Twinkie at all.

GAS AND BUTTER

Twinkies' buttery flavor provides the richness we expect from cake and likely also helps to mask their oiliness. Since due to cost and rancidity issues there's no room in a packaged cake like Twinkies for fresh butter, artificial butter is the answer—the same "butter flavor" used on movie popcorn (what many theaters accurately and nonsensically refer to as "golden-flavored topping") as well as in French vanilla ice cream. The most surprising thing about it is that it really stinks.

One of the most desirable artificial flavors due to its taste and versatility, artificial butter, like many flavor chemicals, smells positively awful in its concentrated state. "Terrible, revolting" is what one expert called it, not an auspicious start. Diacetyl—the "di" in the name refers to its molecular structure, and the "acetyl" part shows that it is related to acetic acid and acetylene welding gas—is so powerfully bad-smelling that some companies that deal with it do so in a dedicated, separate building. But diacetyl is a very common, smooth, slippery, butter/butterscotch flavor, and it occurs naturally quite often in spoiled fruit juice and over-fermented beer. A mere touch of it—it is detectable in concentrations as low as fifty parts per *billion*—gives Chardonnay wine its smoothness;

higher concentrations are what make butter smell like butter, but even higher concentrations are what make butter smell rancid.

Diacetyl could also be extracted from butter, but that is extremely difficult and expensive. It can be fermented from yeast, and sometimes is, but luckily, the same exact molecule is more inexpensively created from natural gas by a few obscure Chinese chemical companies and a well-known German multinational corporation. And once it's baked into a cake, unlike butter, it doesn't need refrigeration. All it takes is the biggest chemical plants in the world, a major dose of petroleum, a little hydrochloric acid, plus some very unexotic and inexpensive water and air.

BASF makes diacetyl and tens of thousands of other chemicals at its headquarters in Ludwigshafen, Germany, smack on the Rhine, a bit south of Frankfurt. Though it is almost a commodity, the actual process used is kept secret, but given the company's massive network of interconnected petrochemical production facilities, BASF probably takes butane, a natural gas component, and processes it with ultrahot steam into a clear, very volatile, flammable liquid called methyl ethyl ketone (MEK), technically the main aroma in blue cheese (try telling that to a French cheesemaker). In fact, it actually smells more like a sweet hospital antiseptic.

You can also buy a can of MEK at hardware stores, in case you want to make diacetyl at home (kids, don't do this!) or, more likely, thin some epoxy resin when repairing your boat or car (kids, don't do this, either). In the final step, when the MEK is passed over a rare metal catalyst like vanadium oxide and then mixed with a little of the basic, common hydrochloric acid, it changes to diacetyl, a volatile liquid that is such a bright, intense, fluorescent yellow that you can easily see where real butter gets its color. Packed carefully into twenty-five-kilogram drums and sealed with a layer of nitrogen to protect it from moisture and fire (it is so highly flammable that a vapor mixture can actually explode) it must be stored under refrigeration. On top of that, due to the strength of its apparently awful (but nontoxic) smell, diacetyl must be kept separate from other chemicals and treated carefully to guard against leaks. The containers are labeled "harmful if swallowed," both ironic and ominous for a food ingredient.

When the flavor houses are finished with diacetyl, it is usually no longer pure. Much as is done with artificial vanilla extract, they buy the pure stuff from one of the big chemical companies and then blend it for a rounder, more useful flavor profile to sell to the food companies. Instead of a dash of salt or a touch of wine, though, they usually add more petroleum products: butyric acid, deltadodecalactone, and propylene glycol (as was used with vanillin). They also might even add vanilla, which is kind of odd when you consider that they're using vanilla to round out a flavor that is used to round out vanilla.

Like politics, food science makes strange bedfellows, mixing odd ingredients and yielding even odder results, and butyric acid takes the cake for odd. This flavor, a natural component of Parmesan cheese, rancid butter, and, unbelievably, vomit and perspiration, is made by passing carbon monoxide, not quite your usual food ingredient (but a great source of carbon and oxygen in a reaction), over a mixture of sodium metal catalysts at 400°F. The result is an oily, colorless, foul-smelling liquid that eventually suggests . . . butter.

A touch of milky, creamy, waxy coconut, and peach or plum notes are added by mixing even more petrochemicals—a bunch of lactones, the most prominent of which has the great, long name deltadodecalactone. This fragrant, translucent yellowish-green, somewhat toxic, highly flammable liquid is handled with special care at the flavor company because, should it spill, the smell would be extraordinarily difficult to clean up. Of course, once it is processed, chemical reactions totally neutralize any toxicity and flammability.

With these unlikely ingredients, Twinkies' butter flavor is created—quite literally—out of gas. It joins the two versions of vanilla and with them evokes or creates those wonderful childhood memories that, in part, drive Twinkies' popularity. Luckily, only a little is needed—the flavors are blended into the batter so artfully by one of the world's best emulsifiers, an ingredient made from two vegetable acids and a caustic liquid that started out as table salt.

- - - - - - - - - - - - - -

CHAPTER 21

Sodium Stearoyl Lactylate

It is hard to say what SSL actually is or what the home equivalent is. And yet, sodium stearoyl lactylate is the ingredient that gives bakers the most bang for their buck. If they had to choose one additive to use in a bakery, it would be SSL (as it's known to the cognoscenti), for its surprisingly multifaceted nature. Whatever it is, exactly, its ingredients come from all over the country, and possibly the South Pacific. And here you thought vanilla was exotic.

TIGHTENING AND WHIPPING UP

Like a good mate, sodium stearoyl lactylate offers both strength and softness, unlike other additives, which are capable of providing only one or the other. In keeping with its tendency to overachieve, SSL starts working before a batter is even baked, acting as a "dough conditioner," stabilizing and strengthening it and improving the protein, simply making it easier to manipulate. Then, both before and during cooking, even though it is more of a fat, SSL functions as an emulsifier instead: it helps to tighten and increase the volume of the crumb, partly by helping to retain the gas created by the leavening. (Think Wonder® Bread as opposed to an airy French baguette.) In coffee whiteners (artificial creamers), puddings, and low-fat margarines it also acts as an emulsifier. It "complexes" the starch, keeping bread softer, longer (this is antistaling; though it is not considered a preservative, SSL certainly helps preserve Twinkies by extending shelf life). Finally, it works as a whipping aid and so creates creaminess in the Twinkie filling (along with polysorbate 60), which is why it is often found in cheese sauces, cream liqueurs, and Hunt's Snack Pack Vanilla Pudding (and in Jell-O® Pudding Snacks, too, emphatically described as being "for smooth texture"). Despite this heroic list of attributes, the powerful SSL remains a minor ingredient, usually less than 1 percent of a flour mixture like Twinkies, making it quite inexpensive.

A totally fabricated additive, it still most closely duplicates the humble egg yolk in home recipes. Food scientists and product developers will tell you (as they repeatedly told me) that SSL is a whole lot better than eggs, and, for that matter, better than Better'n Eggs® (which has no yolks, either). All it takes to make it is some rocks (sodium) from Wyoming, palm trees or soybeans (stearoyl) processed in Massachusetts, corn (lactylate) processed in Nebraska, and a big processing facility in Missouri.

A Dash of Salt?

The first subingredient, which lends the "sodium," to sodium stearoyl lactylate, seems common enough, but in fact turns out to be the one part of the recipe that approaches secret status. That is surprising also because the sodium part of SSL, though listed first in the name, is infinitesimally small. However, it can and often does come from a small dose of soda ash (sodium carbonate)—the same raw material used to make sodium acid pyrophosphate—

such as that mined and processed in Green River, Wyoming, by FMC. Shipped by railcar as a powder or a liquid to SSL manufacturers, the soda ash is unloaded by a giant vacuum or pump and stored in small silos. The sodium can also come from either solid or liquid sodium hydroxide (lye), made from salt as part of the chloralkali process, or even sodium methoxide, a toxic mixture of methanol and sodium hydroxide. For the open-minded scientists at an SSL manufacturing plant, such as American Ingredients in Grandview, Missouri, it makes no difference where the sodium comes from, so they choose based on availability and, of course, price. All the toxic chemicals get rearranged and neutralized in the upcoming reactions, anyway.

Candle Acid

Stearic acid, perhaps from Twin Rivers, in Quincy, Massachusetts, among other places, is the second name-giving ingredient in sodium stearoyl lactylate, and it arrives at the plant solid as a candle.[12] (The "-oyl" suffix indicates that something contains an oil or fatty acid.) On a single, private track in back of American Ingredients' SSL plant, workers patiently pump steam into the outer jackets of a few tank cars in order to liquefy this fully hydrogenated oil, which melts at 170°F. With 160,000 pounds in each car, it takes twelve hours to pump out a tank car, even using a six-inch-wide hose.

The River Effect

In a darkened, quiet area of a sterile pump, pipe, and tank loft of Cargill's corn biorefinery in Blair, Nebraska, where corn

---

12. Candles, soaps, plastics, pastels, lubricants, and cosmetics (such as Vaseline® Intensive Care Dry Skin Lotion) all claim stearic acid as an ingredient, there mostly to add slipperiness and bulk.

sweeteners of all kinds are made by the ton every minute from Midwestern field corn, a nondescript, eight-inch-wide pipe extends through the wall, carrying corn syrup full of sugary dextrose. A white steel truss supports this pipe from the corn syrup plant, across the industrial campus's parking lot, and over to some bright steel towers at the lactic acid plant. The air smells sweet. An old farm's windmill turns slowly in the distance, calling to mind the Netherlands, the headquarters for the world's largest lactic acid manufacturer, Purac, which happens to own the plant I'm about to enter.

Attached to the plant buildings is a solid, new, cement-paneled office building, which looks like it could withstand any form of extreme weather the Great Plains might throw at it. (Later on I learn that my hunch is right; it doubles as a tornado shelter.) The plant manager, a scientist-brewer named Kevin Shoemaker, provides a whiteboard tour of biochemistry via a three-color, thirty-two-box flowchart that he draws from memory. Waypoints on the board tour include fermentation, calcification, biomass separation, swap reaction, dilute lactic acid, purification and concentration, and finally, lactic acid. This is not a walk in the park, or, since we're in rural Nebraska, a stroll in the field.

✳

Lactic acid, the third name-giving ingredient in SSL, is a natural acid, one type of which is made in our bodies by bursts of muscular activity. It is what makes your muscles feel sore and tired and gives you cramps in your side when you're running. (It seems appropriate to reflect on this as I climb up and around the lactic acid plant and feel the burn in my thighs.) It also occurs naturally due to the fermentation of sugar in foods ranging from sauerkraut to meat. Lactic acid is responsible for the sour taste in spoiled milk and the sour taste in cheese (and Cheetos® too). Unsurprisingly, its name comes from the Latin word *lack*, meaning "milk." Carl

Wilhelm Scheele, the great Swedish chemist, first isolated lactic acid from sour milk in 1780, and this former waste product has been used to make food ever since. But the lactic acid made for food use, for use in Twinkies, is not made from milk—it's made from dextrose, a corn syrup.

Lactic acid, like salt, brings out savory flavors in beverages and foods and, as such, has long been used as a preservative in processed meat and poultry. While helping to enhance flavor, it also stabilizes and preserves salad dressings. It extends shelf life and helps fix the color of pickles, olives, and other brined vegetables. On the sweet side, it is a staple of hard candy and fruit gum. It is a natural sourdough acid, and, of course, it plays a role in cake recipes, too, either as an acid itself, or, as with Twinkies, as part of the versatile emulsifier SSL.

Lactic acid is utilized in a number of fascinating and totally unpredictable ways in industry, too, ranging from tanning leather to making CD ROMs. And it is made from renewable resources. Purac seems to have found a good business to be in; its parent company reports sales of $5 billion a year.

✳

Outside, the dextrose pipe from the corn syrup plant leads to the fermenters, a small group of closed, cylindrical towers, each about one story high, surrounded by a mass of pipes and valves. First, the dextrose is piped into the towers along with a little benign bacteria to start the fermentation, just like yeast is used to make beer (as with beer, the choice of bacteria is key, and here, it's top secret). In one corner stands a little silo, from which lime is fed in with the bacteria as needed to control the fermentation's pH level. The lime is likely to come from the Mississippi Lime Company, the same place that supplies it to many other food processors for items like monocalcium phosphate.

The result is a nice broth of calcium lactate (the product of the calcification stage), and, as is fitting, the first tank it is piped into is called the "broth surge tank." Here the biomass created by the fermentation, the spent bacteria, becomes a useful waste product, as the crunchy, dry leftover is separated from the liquid—spun out in a centrifuge operation—ground up slightly, and in a nifty bit of true recycling, sold to local farmers as a nitrogen and phosphorus-rich fertilizer for corn. Brewers are always known to gardeners and farmers for their great waste products, and it's no different here in Nebraska.

Next, sulfuric acid, one of the most common basic chemicals, is channeled through polypropylene-lined pipes for a quick "swap" reaction with the calcium that creates calcium sulfate, better known as gypsum, which is then precipitated out, along with every trace of sulfuric acid. Shoemaker reaches into a steel machine to grab a handful for me to feel. With the consistency of wet sand, this by-product is sold wet, locally, as a soil amendment, which makes sense for everyone, as it is more easily taken up by the soil that way, and would be costly to dry.

What's left is dilute lactic acid, which travels through a series of concentration tanks and a forest of forty-foot-tall, ten-foot-wide, white, cylindrical, steam-heated evaporators for purification. The first few concentration tanks are linked heat exchangers known as effects. Looking something like a four-story-high, front-loading washing machine, the porthole at the bottom of each offers a clear view of the acid drying. What started out as a brown milk shake is now a clear, almost watery syrup.

Shoemaker interrupts the quality control lab momentarily to land me a sample of lactic acid. The startled technicians rummage around, and after ten or so seconds come up with a bottle of what looks to be water. It is too concentrated to taste, but just right for sniffing. "Sort of a mild sweet and sour?" I ask, hoping to get it right. "With a bit of caramel," Shoemaker adds. A caramel note, indeed. "What do you think, Tony?" Shoemaker asks a young lab tech. I half expect him to say something like, "The 2002 had much more oaki-ness, with a hint of fruit," but instead he replies, "Kinda sweet."

No oak barrels for this wine. From the tank loft the fresh acid is pumped outside into a small farm of holding tanks, and then into a loading bay where stainless steel tank trucks and big black tank railcars stand ready to run it downriver to Grandview, Missouri, where it will be made into sodium stearoyl lactylate, along with the two other unlikely cake-mates.

Blowing Hot and Cold

Posters outlining the steps of how to brew complex Belgian beers line the walls of one scientist's office at American Ingredients, part of the company that held the original patent on sodium stearoyl lactylate, from the early 1950s, and now one of the few specialized enough to make it. Beer brewing is food chemistry, too, though the process is slightly older, by thousands or tens of thousands of years. It also presents quite a contrast to the stainless steel–clad, computer-driven alchemy that the company works with—one step in the Belgian beer-brewing process calls for it to sit in open vats in old, spider- and dust-laden barns. We certainly won't see *that* with any Twinkie ingredients.

The prairie wind blasts the plant (the same one that makes mono and diglycerides) but doesn't disturb its compact tank farm, the smallest of which holds an intriguing substance: liquid nitrogen. The valves at the bottom are frozen in ice piles several feet high, despite the sun, because what's inside is chilled to 350 degrees *below* zero Fahrenheit. A huge radiator, ten feet tall and twenty feet wide, warms it a bit en route to the plant so that it gasifies. This way it can be used as a blanket in the storage and processing tanks, driving out the oxygen and keeping these precious food fluids fresh.

Troy Boutté, American's Director of Research and Development, is again my guide. Boutté helps me trace the pipes that carry both the stearic acid and the lactic acid inside and into stainless steel reactor vessels, each the size of a delivery truck. The mixer motors in each kettle are grinding away full tilt. The kettles are so big that it takes about six hours to fill them; the mix cooks for only about two hours. Bursts of steam punctuate the atmosphere while heating the giant kettles. A small shot of the sodium material—a soupçon of sodium carbonate or a similar alkali (whatever it is remains unidentified by my guides)—brings the reaction to a halt. Any caustic qualities are immediately neutralized by the base's reaction with the two acids (stearic and lactic), which are themselves quite gentle. The result is a gentle yet fabulously useful salt, but at this point it is a hot, thick, fatty syrup, a white glop that is pumped over a slowly rotating ten-foot-diameter, stainless steel drum called a "flaker."

I'm surprised to find that the flaker isn't hot, given that a dry powder is the goal. In fact, it doesn't dry the mixture—it actually cools it, so that it solidifies in a matter of seconds on the chilled drum surface, much as candle wax solidifies on your finger. It tastes like it looks, and that's not good: soapy wax. No surprise: soap is a salt of a fatty acid; sodium stearate is a common soap ingredient, and I've just inadvertently put some in my mouth, bringing back memories of childhood punishments. I begin to wonder about my taste buds recovering, and how Twinkies succeed in absorbing this taste (hint: there's only a touch of it in the batter).

The opaque wax dries clear. As the drum rotates, a long blade fixed against it, the waxy stuff is scraped off and allowed to fall in a snowy cascade. I look down to see a snowbank of sparkling flakes, some reflecting light like the mica that sparkles so dazzlingly under streetlights during a nighttime snow shower, providing a delicate angle to this machinery-laden scene.

The newly broken flakes then fall one story down, through a

ten-foot-wide funnel, only to be conveyed back up four stories to a grinder, then dropped back down into a large, vibrating tub called a classifier, which is filled with screen sieves so that only the desired powder falls into the fifty-pound, plastic-bag-lined boxes below it. Boutté and I head across the steel grates and down to the next level of humming machines to snag a sample, which is indescribably fluffy, a superfine powder that coats my hands instantly. It is almost impossible to wipe off, but since it's soluble, it washes off easily (and blends into batter really well).

Each box is filled with a whoosh and sent on its way down the roller conveyor to be shipped out. And we're shipping out, too. I've got soapy SSL on my taste buds and dinner on my mind, grateful that Kansas City's famed barbecue is only minutes away. I just hope that there's no sodium stearoyl lactylate in the barbecue sauce.

Sodium steroyl lactylate is fascinating because it is manufactured mostly from things you would never eat, like soda ash or stearic acid or field corn, and it largely duplicates the role played by egg yolks. You don't need it at home. At least sodium caseinate, which is made from at least one toxic raw material, originates primarily from a familiar and tasty raw material—milk.

CHAPTER 22

Sodium and Calcium Caseinate

The very best casein, the protein part of milk that usually gets made into cheese, comes from the Waikato region of New Zealand, an area described to me by a New Zealand trade emissary as *Lord of the Rings* land. It doesn't come from the United States, that's for sure. No American dairy can afford to process casein into caseinates, the least profitable part of milk. U.S. dairies much prefer to transform milk into more profitable cheese, which also leads to the very profitable sweet dairy whey. But then we go and import well over 200 million pounds of casein each year to make Twinkies and a host of other food products, despite our being the largest dairy-producing country in the world. Let's hope that the cows of Belarus graze upwind of Chernobyl, because Belarus, along with Russia and Poland, is where a lot of the cheaper milk we use to make lower grades of sodium and calcium caseinate comes from.

Lucky for us, New Zealand and Ireland (our two biggest suppliers by far), where the most expensive milk comes from, don't turn all their milk into beverages or cheese, hence the endless supply of casein. There, caseinates are made directly from fresh milk;

elsewhere the milk is dried first and has to be rehydrated back into milk once it's imported here—a seemingly unnecessary and rather unpalatable extra step. They also work within various and complex trade agreements (and loopholes in GATT, apparently) to facilitate dairy exports. New Zealand is the world's largest casein exporter, half of which goes to the United States.[13]

REMEMBER THE ALAMO!

In the late 1800s, casein was used to make "milk paint," something house restorers today curse still as they struggle to remove it; it was also made into glue, which might explain the paint's tenacity, something old house restorers can certainly relate to (it is still used in latex paints). Casein helped form the first plastics, in the late 1800s and early 1900s, when it was mixed with formaldehyde and hardened into pens, buckles, and knife handles; casein buttons were the norm at the turn of the twentieth century, made into imitation tortoiseshell, jade, and lapis lazuli. (It was certainly not considered a food ingredient back then.)

Major domestic production stopped as far back as the 1950s. Then, casein had long been treated as something of a waste product, being part of the skim milk left over from butter-making or excess curds from cheese-making. Much as with whey, now another valuable food additive also found in Twinkies, it was often used for pig feed or simply tossed out. And wouldn't you know it, around that time the big food companies spearheaded a hunt for food additives that would increase shelf life and extend the usefulness of, or replace, traditional ingredients such as eggs and

---

13. Small change is in the air, however, and domestic casein production might well begin again. The USDA has or had what appears to be a small, secret program to sell some surplus dried milk to several U.S. companies that can make caseinates, but has some kind of gag order and is not forthcoming with details.

milk. A dried milk component—dried milk had been on the scene for years—was an obvious candidate to explore as a possible functional ingredient. And it turned out to be high in protein, making it nutritious.

Until the 1950s, Borden®, of Elsie the Cow fame, had used casein to make Elmer's glue and paste for elementary school children. (That was the paste you could eat, at least technically, because it was made from milk. That paste is no longer around, though some argue it was simply moved to the cafeteria.) And that's not the only reason Borden's is a memorable part of American culture and history. Gail Borden Jr., who invented canned milk in 1856 (and put an eagle on his brand of sweetened condensed milk, the one that remains on market shelves to this day), made a fortune during the Civil War. But he has a more dramatic claim to fame: in 1835, he founded a small newspaper, the *Telegraph and Texas Register*, in Galveston (which he also helped lay out and found) before becoming a dairyman in New York State. Borden's paper was one of the first to report on the Texans' battles for independence from Mexico. His March 1836 headline helped to immortalize the famous battle cry, "Remember the Alamo!" The (temporarily) victorious Mexicans responded by throwing his printing press into a river and may have thereby convinced Borden to focus on canned milk instead of politics, much to our collective benefit.

Nutrition and Whipped Toppings

Caseinate, whether sodium or calcium, is a top source of protein, and rich in the eight essential amino acids. Eighty percent of the protein in milk can be found in the casein (the rest is in the whey). While nutritional value is helpful if you are making an energy bar or protein-fortified meal replacement drink—both caseinates are in Nutrament® "energy and fitness drink" and Slim-Fast Optima™—it is less important if you are baking, say, a snack cake like a Twinkie. In fact, there is no home equivalent for this white powder other than milk itself. (You don't really need sodium caseinate unless you make your own sausages, and then it makes a strong binder when powdered milk just won't do. Sausage makers used dried milk for years—as did cake bakers like Hostess—before modern technology brought us sodium caseinate.)

In Twinkies, proteins aren't there to promote strong bodies. Caseinates, especially sodium caseinate, work mainly in the filling, emulsifying, stabilizing, gelling, and absorbing a little water. Though definitely minor players, they nonetheless play an essential role in keeping that filling aerated and just a little bit foamy.

They play a more important role, however, in many other foods. Caseinates help make dough uniform in mass-produced doughnuts, muffins, and waffles, and block the excess absorption of fat in fried foods. They emulsify and stabilize packaged milk shake/drink bases; carry flavors and minimize shrinkage in ice cream and other frozen desserts like Breyers® Carb Smart Ice Cream Bars; bind and emulsify fat in processed meats (sausage, luncheon meat); and clarify wine (fine particles coagulate with the protein in casein and are easily filtered out). Caseinates help extend eggs (whole, white, or yolk), they support meringue and other foods made of egg whites, and form the films on edible glazes. They also add some authenticity to synthetic milk additives (they are rather important in coffee creamers like Coffeemate®), stickiness to edible adhesives, and, being dairy products, a bit of legitimacy to analog (fake) cheese, which can be made from not much more than sodium caseinate, flavor, salt, stabilizers, and water, though a more complex version, based on soy, includes casein too (Veggie Slices® Cheese Alternative American Flavor Organic). Low in calories and high in nutrients, caseinates function well as fat replacers.

The most fascinating industrial role casein plays is in making concrete. Part of a new system of products that reduce the amount of water needed so much that the curing time is cut by half, casein is saving oodles of money for builders. And in keeping with its historical tasks, casein is also used in high-end furniture glue. With a long list like that, casein has come a long way since elementary school paste.

White Powder into White Powder

In New Zealand and Ireland, milk is converted to dried caseinate right at the dairy. A bit of hydrochloric acid (instead of an enzyme like rennet) separates milk into curds and whey, only this time the curds get made into Twinkies and energy drinks instead of cheese.

The process is actually pretty simple. Washing curds with a dilute alkali solution, made either with a sodium solution (this would be sodium hydroxide, or lye, again) for sodium caseinate, or a lime solution (calcium hydroxide, or lime) for calcium caseinate, neutralizes the acid milk product, making it into a more useful salt. After the wash, the caseinate solutions are spray-dried— atomized under high pressure into a stainless steel spray-drying chamber that can be as much as five stories high and 375°F hot. There, the liquid caseinate hits the heat and instantly drops to the bottom of the chamber as a fine, pale yellow powder, ready for packaging and shipping to bakeries. The big plants in New Zealand can top an astounding thirty thousand pounds per hour doing this. The process may be simple, but the volume is high.

Because powdered minerals—calcium and sodium—are mixed with caseinates, they essentially become dairy products. Not so with the last mineral on the list, calcium sulfate. Almost nothing happens to it.

CHAPTER 23

Calcium Sulfate

Here's yet another rock that we eat, and it comes from only one place in the country. In spite of its chemical name, and in spite of the fact that its sister product, plaster of Paris, is used to make casts and walls—two decidedly uncakelike items (depending on who's doing the cooking)—calcium sulfate shares the distinction (with eggs, salt, and water) of being the least processed of Twinkie ingredients. We hardly do anything to it before eating it. Like salt, it comes from an ancient marine deposit near the earth's surface, and like salt, it is essential to our health.

OKLAHOMA OCEAN

Although gypsum is one of the most common minerals in the world, nowhere else is it found—and used—in such quantities as in the United States, and most is found in Oklahoma. The purest gypsum, the only gypsum approved for use in food, is found in the northwestern quadrant of Oklahoma, in a rolling area called the Gypsum Hills that sparkles with glasslike crystals. Canyons in nearby Gloss Mountain State Park (sometimes called Glass Mountain—the name was apparently given by an upper-crust Brit whose strong accent disguised his intent) show dramatic layers of white rock alternating with red earth. Even the earth is calcium enriched.

Rising not-so-grandly 150 to 200 feet above the nearby Red Beds Plains area farmland, many of these small hills are—or rather, were, until they were quarried—capped by layers of gypsum five to eighteen feet thick. In the tiny town of Southard, just northwest of Oklahoma City, the United States Gypsum company (USG), makers of the familiar wallboard, Sheetrock®, operates the quarry that yields just about all of our food-grade calcium sulfate.

USG and a nearby, small competitor mining the same vein, Allied Custom Gypsum, use this source for agricultural and industrial gypsum products, too—only about 5 percent of the rock is used for food. The same gypsum deposit covers much of the central United States, another Twinkie ingredient (like salt, limestone, and phosphates) laid down hundreds of millions of years ago by an expanded Pacific Ocean. Where the gypsum approaches the surface there are now mines or quarries and wallboard facilities (and towns like Gypsum, Ohio; Gypsum, Colorado; and Plaster City, California; Southard, Oklahoma, is an exception, being named after the first miner here, George Franklin Southard).

Though known as a mineral in your diet, calcium is actually a so-called earth metal, like sodium, and a reactive one, too—it is always found attached to something else. In this case, it is found attached to sulfur and mixed with water—and, in addition to being called gypsum, it's known as hydrous calcium sulfate, or calcium sulfate dihydrate. (The "di" means that there are two molecules of water attached to each calcium sulfate molecule.) You might find calcium deposit in your own home, especially if you have hard well water (though this would be calcium carbonate, not sulfate) in the form of a white crust left behind after you've boiled water. There's a reason the word "gypsum" is derived from *gypsos*, Greek for "chalk."

Plaster is made by cooking gypsum just right. Heating it ever so gently removes about three-fourths of the gypsum's natural water so that it absorbs water eagerly when mixed on a construction site (some lime and silica are usually added by the manufacturers to delay setting or to add surface hardness). After this simple processing, gypsum wins the honor of being the only rock that can be crushed into a powder and then turned back into a rock just by adding water. That's why you can make plaster out of it (but not Twinkies). The calcium sulfate used in food looks and feels like plaster, and, scarily, even solidifies when wet, but is not as strong (I know, I tried it in my office).

Calcium sulfate has a riveting history. Though plaster was used on the ancient Egyptian pyramids and Greek temples, it was the French who popularized it as plaster of Paris (duh). Paris sits on top of a major gypsum deposit, and old gypsum quarries exist beneath much of the city, including under the Notre Dame cathedral.

According to legend, Benjamin Franklin is responsible for the success of plaster of Paris as a soil amendment in the United States (it promotes aeration in clay soils). He was our first ambassador to France, and so admired its use while he was there that he brought some back here in 1785. An energetic promoter, he worked it into the soil on a prominent hillside in the form of letters reading, THIS HAS BEEN PLASTERED. When the clover growing over the enriched soil grew dramatically denser than the analphabetic clover around it, he had successfully introduced gypsum as "land plaster" to American farmers. (The strange thing is that ancient Greeks gardened with it, too, so it is not clear why Franklin's coaxing seemed new to the Americans.) Imported from Paris at first, gypsum's popularity was assured when deposits were found in abundance around the United States.

Plaster of Paris was always a popular wall finish, of course, but plaster is hard to use on walls without talent and time, a big problem for Americans. In the 1880s, a man named Augustine Sackett figured out how to dry a layer of plaster between two pieces of thick paper, inventing gypsum wallboard. It really took off on a national scale when his Sheetrock® was featured at the 1933 Chicago World's Fair. Now it seems that every wall is made of it. And the gypsum producers are glad to add cooking to calcium sulfate's vast array of industrial uses. But for food, it must be pure.

TWINKIES AND TOFU

Calcium sulfate wasn't officially approved for food use in the States until January 1980. But we're way behind the rest of the world in that way. Gypsum has been used in food for more than two thousand years, though not for Twinkies.

In China, gypsum was used during the Han dynasty for coagulating soy milk to make tofu; some say it may have been used to stiffen bread dough in King David's Jerusalem. Flour that is low in calcium can produce soft, sticky dough that would frustrate any ancient or modern baker and would be a nightmare for the major bakeries with all their pumps and machines; that's why calcium sulfate is found in most types of regular bread. (Commercial bakers need more of a flowing batter rather than a stiff, dry dough, so any stiffness is relative.) Added in minute percentages—never more than 1.3 percent by law—calcium sulfate is loosely categorized as a dough conditioner for baked goods, its most common food function. But that description is very limiting. Some suppliers have identified more than one hundred uses for calcium sulfate as a direct food additive. And it is as cheap as common salt.

The main thing calcium sulfate does sometimes is take up space. In Twinkies, it also acts as a filler, keeping the custom-mixed baking powder ingredients mixed evenly and preventing caking, which is what it does in Kraft® Calumet® Double-Acting Baking Powder (same as cornstarch does in other brands)—perhaps the only way calcium sulfate finds its way onto your kitchen shelf. In short, you don't need it at home, and you can't buy it at the store.

Calcium sulfate also acts as an economical nutrient, adding a considerable amount of calcium to foods like Wonder® Bread (20 percent of your daily value) at a bargain price. Calcium sulfate may also be the reason Twinkies can claim to provide a percent daily value of calcium per cake, but only as a beneficial by-product of its more important function in the batter. It works as a nutrient in soy cheeses, feeds yeast, and balances the acidity in cakes. And calcium sulfate helps canned fruits and vegetables retain firmness and stay juicy by binding with natural pectin and increasing their water-holding capacity.

Beer brewers use calcium sulfate to raise pH, and to control proteins and starches to get a paler, smoother-tasting, more stable beer that lasts longer on the shelf. It clarifies brewing water, too, in case a brewer doesn't have a pure Rocky Mountain spring to draw from. And it fills out pharmaceuticals, while supplying a little extra calcium to boot, even though it is not an active ingredient. The totally dry version, a filler favored by pill makers, is so white (with the inevitable brand name of Snow White®, of course) that it is sometimes used to make cake icings whiter. Natural food stores allow calcium sulfate in their stocks when it is used as a moisture absorbent and filler in capsules of other nutritional supplements. On the industrial side, calcium sulfate is added to plastic coatings, adhesives, and grouts for extra strength and reduced shrinkage. Quikcrete®, ready-mixed patching cement, even includes a good dose of the Snow White filler for a clean, professional finish.

Calcium sulfate is cheap and plentiful, odorless, nontoxic, and tasteless. It does a good job at just over 1 percent of a recipe. Even at these low doses, we somehow manage to consume an astounding twenty-eight pounds each over a lifetime. What's amazing is how little we have to do to it in order to eat it. Unlike plaster of Paris, the calcium sulfate destined for food escapes the oven altogether. What you eat is basically what is dug out of the ground. It's just easier to chew than solid rock because it's been ground into a superfine white powder.

Scrape and Grind

The gypsum at the Southard quarry is as pure as it comes: 98 to 99 percent (the food laws require 98 percent). Famous for its purity since George Southard staked his claim and opened it in the first few years of the twentieth century, Dave Hollingshead, the current quarry manager, keeps busy "knocking the tops off the hills," as he puts it. After removing as much as seventy-five feet of hilltop made of brown surface soil and rocks (mostly shale) with earthmoving equipment, meticulous workers use mechanical brooms and scrapers to make the bright white rock clean of any soil. Now that USG is no longer blasting the stuff out of the ground with dynamite, and mines were phased out in the 1940s, Hollingshead's crews carefully scrape four inches of the white rock at a pass into neat windrows with what look like road planers, giant vehicles with rotating sharp blades beneath their chassis. Superclean front-loaders scoop up fist-size chunks as well as smaller granules and dump them into clean trucks that carry them quickly over company-built roads to the nearby mill for crushing. Any impure rock can be made into wallboard, but pure calcium sulfate makes superior plaster.

There's enough pure calcium sulfate here to last until about 2030. The mine pits are usually the size of a few football fields and scattered over seven thousand acres, an area roughly ten miles long and a couple miles wide. Mounds of white rock surround the crushing plant, an agglomeration of mostly low-slung, steel buildings connected by a half dozen hundred-foot-long, elevated, angled conveyors. Against the earth tones of its surroundings, the bright white rock contrasts nicely. Here the chunks are reduced to the size of sugar or salt crystals in circular crushers called Raymond mills, thick rings of cast iron with interior rollers that fling themselves constantly against the inside. The particles are then screened, milled repeatedly, fine-screened, passed over by magnets, and finally air-separated from plain rocks and other debris to make a fine powder that behaves like well-sifted flour, which is essential, since much of it is premixed with flour for baking. As if this were some kind of rite of passage, only after the gypsum is ground can it be called by its food-grade name, terra alba, Latin for "white earth."

The calcium sulfate destined for use as a filler, whether for food, pharmaceuticals, or paint, is an even finer powder that is calcined, or dried, to the point of complete dehydration, accomplished by passing it through a continuous oven. (Plaster was made for decades in a much more dramatic way by "boiling" the rock powder in a series of ten-foot-high and wide kettles to the point where you could literally see steam coming out.) Each batch of calcium sulfate processed for food use is measured by atomic absorption analysis, tested and certified for purity before being bagged or loaded into a truck or railcar and sent off to the bakeries. Like so many Twinkies ingredients, both grades are kosher. All of the steps taken with food-grade calcium sulfate are simple and limited to mechanical processes so that calcium sulfate earns a "natural" label from the folks in Washington who examine such things. Then again, it's just a rock.

Simple, useful, inexpensive. Ben Franklin would have loved it ("A penny saved is a penny earned"), although it is not clear if he would have loved Twinkies. And he never could have imagined making a preservative like sorbic acid from petroleum, definitely not.

CHAPTER 24

Sorbic Acid

Twinkies, so fabled for their longevity, in fact contain only one preservative: sorbic acid.

All those myths about Twinkies having an infinite shelf life and being made solely of chemicals are not only wrong, but way, way off. Sure, the chemicals contained in many of the prior ingredients give it a longer shelf life, but they don't actually preserve Twinkies—they mostly retain moisture, prolong softness, fight staling, and replace expensive, spoilable, naturally moist ingredients like butter, milk, and eggs. But cakes still need perfectly airtight plastic wrappers to stay "fresh" (remove the wrapper and the Twinkie is toast, turning hard as rock in no time). Sorbic acid doesn't help with any of those things.

The most persnickety enemy of anything moist is mold, and the best thing around to fight mold is sorbic acid. What's very, very reassuring is that sorbic acid is undramatically, boringly safe—so safe, it actually qualifies as a food itself. The only worrisome thing about it? How it is made—and that, it turns out, is a far cry from food processing.

OIL AND VINEGAR

I had visions of locating the people who harvest some kind of berries to extract sorbic acid from, but, unsurprisingly, no one makes it from natural sources anymore. If you want to keep mold off Twinkies, you'd do a lot better with organic chemistry than a bunch of berries. Despite actually being a food, sorbic acid is made from petroleum. Nutrinova in Frankfurt, Germany, Daicel Chemical Industries in Arai, Japan, and Nantong Acetic Acid Chemical Co. in the Yangtze River valley of China—the only major makers of sorbic acid—make it from natural gas they import from Russia or Norway, the Asian Pacific, or China, respectively. Clearly this is not a local chemical. Not one berry is harmed in the making of these cakes.

I could say that sorbic acid is made from crotanaldehyde (let's call it C) and diketene (let's call it D), but that wouldn't be doing you any favors. Neither one is a familiar chemical. Creating sorbic acid is complicated, which is probably why each company's recipe is confidential and visitors are not welcome despite earnest and persistent efforts. Major chemical plants and oil refineries are not commonly open to scrutiny. But the science is out there if you dig deep enough.

The two main ingredients start with natural gas, cracked to make ethane gas (for C) and methane gas (for D). The ethane then becomes ethylene oxide, the same as is used for polysorbate 60. With the help of palladium, a rare form of platinum, this gas becomes C, a clear, stinky, and flammable liquid.

At the same time, the methane transforms into methanol (wood alcohol) with a little help from carbon monoxide. (Yes, *that* carbon monoxide! But don't worry—it is not an ingredient, just a convenient source of chemicals that become part of a complex reaction . . . the same way it is used to keep your supermarket ground beef looking fresh. You did know that, didn't you?) That methanol is then reacted again with more carbon monoxide to make acetic acid (no, it doesn't come from wine), which itself is "cracked" at 1,300°F to make ketene, a flammable, toxic gas used to make aspirin (go figure), and which is quickly turned into D, a colorless or light yellow and, for once, stable liquid.

When both subingredients C and D are ready, they are mixed with a manganese catalyst (another rare metal—mostly used in steelmaking but also in gasoline mixtures to reduce knocking) to make sugarlike crystals. In China, workers donning lab coats and surgical hats control the processing in twenty-foot-high, bright blue, cylindrical, pressurized vessels from which pipes carry the crystals to tall stainless steel holding tanks that resemble those that you might find in your local microbrewery. They grind the crystals into a fine powder for bakeries and pack them in small, fifty-pound boxes—nothing larger is needed because sorbic acid is so potent. (At this point some caustic potash, potassium hydroxide, or calcium might be mixed in to turn the crystals into the water-soluble, salt versions, potassium sorbate or calcium sorbate—the sister products found in drinks, cheese, and sauces.) Though the whole process definitely does not suggest food, these crystals turns out to be the very benign sorbic acid, harmless and ready to eat.

Safer than Salt

Sorbic acid and its half-sisters, potassium and calcium sorbate, are, inarguably, the most popular preservatives in the world. They are incredibly effective at protecting food against a whole host of evildoers, and manage to do so without killing us in the process. To wit: sorbic acid is less toxic than table salt, so safe that the FDA classifies it as "generally regarded as safe" (GRAS). It is one of the few additives that is legal worldwide.

Bill Riha, Head of Regulatory and Scientific Affairs at Nutri-nova, which makes the majority of sorbic acid, says that despite its completely industrial origin, it is a polyunsaturated, fatty acid akin to soy, olive, or corn oil (sorbic is a "free" short-chain fatty acid, close cousin to the long-chain fatty acids such as those found in olive oil). Its structure is so familiar to our bodies that allergic reactions are extremely rare. The body metabolizes it just like any other fatty acid by turning the sorbic acid into carbon dioxide and water. That may be why even the arch-keen watchdog Center for Science in the Public Interest (CSPI) lists it as safe. And despite being produced by modern technology, the idea of a preservative is rooted in history.

THE DRUID'S STAFF AND ITS UNRIPE BERRY

Since time immemorial, Old World mythology and folklore led humans to believe that the European Rowan, or mountain ash tree (*Sorbus aucuparia*), with its bright orange berries, was magical. It was said to protect against malevolent beings and ward off evil influences, earning the nickname "Thor's Helper," and encouraging voyagers to carry bits of the wood with them for protection against witches. Nowadays, with a little help from oil refineries in Germany and Japan, a synthetic version of a chemical found in those berries protects Twinkies and most other processed foods against malevolent microbes—our modern version of evil influences, at least as far as food is concerned. Sorbic acid takes its name from the mountain ash tree genus, *Sorbus*, which is a big improvement on its real name, trans,trans–2, 4-hexadienoic acid.

Back in 1859, German chemist A. W. Hoffman cooked up a batch of oil distilled from the juice of pressed, unripe mountain ash berries and managed to isolate sorbic acid for the first time (along with some sugars, then called sorbin and sorbit, and even some sorbitol). Apparently, the berries manufacture sorbic acid to protect themselves, resulting in some medicinal qualities. Mountain ash berries proper are too astringent to eat, but their fresh juice or tea has been used as a laxative, a cure for sore throats, inflamed tonsils, and hoarseness, perhaps because it is loaded with vitamin C; jam and infusions made from the berries have been popular remedies for a host of other ailments, including diarrhea, indigestion, hemorrhoids, scurvy, and gout. While I found no record of traditional use of the berries as a preservative, I did come across a mention of their use to make wine, which, in light of some of the berries' above-noted digestive-tract medicinal talents, seems like an astonishingly bad idea.

Rowan branches have often been the choice for dowsing rods and magic wands, as well as Native American bows and arrows. Better than that, though, between its reputation for protection and its natural density, the wood has long been a common material for shafts of all kinds, including walking sticks and druids' staffs.

Only with the advent of the petrochemical industry around 1900 was sorbic acid first synthesized. Still, despite the natural evidence, no one determined for sure its antimicrobial qualities until 1939, when, coincidently, two different scientists—one in Germany and one in the United States—discovered them simultaneously. It was bad timing for the Germans, so Americans naturally took the lead, even netting a patent in 1945. We don't make it in the United States anymore—like so much of our chemical production, it is now solely manufactured abroad. The world's largest producer, Nutrinova, née Hoechst AG, is based in Germany, in an ironic twist of history, though presently it is owned by the giant American global chemical conglomerate Celanese.

LET YOUR KIDS EAT CAKE

It just doesn't seem like sorbic acid is something we should strive to feed our children, and as far as I can tell, there's no home equivalent, either. However, in a nice bit of synergy, it turns out that the reason I don't need a preservative in cakes I make at home is precisely *because* of my kids: they eat them before they can spoil. So kids really do fill a practical function, after all. The proof: about a week after I took some plastic-wrapped, homemade sponge cake to my office, it was green with mold. Moral: keep your cake at home where it can be appreciated. Or use sorbic acid.

Humankind has been preserving food since the start of civilization. Cooking, drying, salting, and smoking were the only options for thousands of years, with fermentation (technically, lactic acid fermentation) added to the mix awhile ago—think cheese and yogurt. We've preserved food over the ages by soaking things in sugar (jam), vinegar (pickles), or alcohol (fruit). But it wasn't until the industrial revolution of the 1800s that we came close to the modern options we have today.

Sorbic acid works in a tremendously complex manner that is not fully understood: essentially, though, we know that a whole bunch of different enzymes work together to stop bacteria and fungus growth (it's classified as a "wide-spectrum antimicrobial"). Try as the bakers might to make snack cakes without water, it's necessary, especially in the filling. With moisture comes the risk of mold (just think of your bathtub), and sorbic acid does the job of preventing it beautifully in a variety of products, including cosmetics and topical ointments. The only thing sorbic acid *does* in a Twinkie is preserve; manufacturers who add the phrase "to preserve freshness" or "as a preservative" to their labels are within the law but could save themselves the space on the ingredient label.

At typical usage levels, you can't smell or taste sorbic acid, even in bland foods, despite its having a slight acid taste and sour odor in concentrated form. Plus, it is strong stuff, used only to the tune of two-tenths of 1 percent of a batch of dough, making an expensive ingredient economical (sometimes it is only 0.03 percent of the food). That's barely three ounces per hundred pounds, a mere dusting. Sorbic acid is, in fact, the stealth additive, true to its mysterious origins.

From berries to bakeries, via refineries. So safe and strong, the next-to-last item on the ingredient list, so little of it is needed. The only ingredients that there are less of in a Twinkie are colors, and they, too, are totally man-made.

CHAPTER 25

FD&C Yellow No. 5, Red No. 40

The last ingredient I explore on my journey is in St. Louis, Missouri, home of the world's largest food color factory: colors are the last item on many ingredient lists, including Twinkies'. A one-ton, Volkswagen-size supersack of powdered, gray acid sits near another supersack of powdered gray salt, both looking as plain and innocuous as can be. A worker mixes some of each into a 5,500-gallon stainless steel vessel called a coupling tank, a name that reflects its odd job of marrying various molecules with new bonds. He adds some clear water, some brown liquid (sodium nitrite—the salt of nitrous acid) as a catalyst, and a little sodium hydroxide (lye) to neutralize the acids, and voilà! Red No. 40. Candy-apple red, with a nice pink foam, a tanker truckload of color that is completely without taste or smell.

A few yards away sit two more supersacks containing the same salt and a similar but unnamed powder. They are mixed in the same way, but the results appear dark brown. Voilà! Raw Yellow No. 5. Turns out that the brightest and strongest food colors are made from dull gray powders and common chemicals.

Welcome to Sensient Colors Inc. On an open steel grate floor, suspended in the air, acids, bases, and salts are mixed carefully to create food dyes. Measurement reminders are taped to the computers: so many inches of this, so many meters of that. Kelly Walsh, a supervisor, opens the inspection hatch of one for a better look (hold on to your glasses!). Big agitator paddles stir the liquid, creating foam on top. Over the next few days Walsh will pump it out—hot, so it doesn't crystallize—and around this room of pipes, valves, and vats to be mixed, filtered, further reacted, purified, and then dried in a six-story-high spray dryer, where it is atomized so that when it hits the extremely hot walls it instantly bounces off as a powder. Powdered color.

BLAND IS BAD

We've been coloring our food since 5000 BC. Even the ancient Romans recognized that "we eat with our eyes," often using saffron, spinach, caramel, and spices to enhance the appearance of their foods. Yellow has been added to butter as far back as the 1300s (possibly saffron, but definitely marigolds), a precursor to our rather strange modern desire for orange cheese. Recipes, whether at home or at the Ritz, specify vegetables and fruit by color, from a simple tomato and mozzarella salad with a sprig of basil to a fancy kiwi tart decorated with a single strawberry. We treasure roasts with rich, dark skins.

Sometimes we expect strong color where natural color is actually weak, which may explain why Ocean Spray includes Red No. 40 in its Ruby Red Grapefruit Juice. At Sensient, color scientists repeatedly state that we taste with our eyes before we taste with our mouths. In Australia, an ice cream company found that it sold three times as much passion fruit ice cream tinted with the pink of the fruit than a plain white version of the exact same ice cream (taste was not affected). In Twinkies sponge cake, perhaps the dark orange color—the mixture of red and yellow—is meant to suggest richness, or lots of butter and eggs (of which we now know there is not). Except for when Hostess colored the filling green for a *Shrek* movie tie-in (yellow mixed with Blue No. 1, about as unappetizing as you can get), Twinkies colors work simply to make the cake *look* like fresh cake. The Larousse Gastronomique sums up food colorings aptly: "Their function is essentially a psychological one."

A Twinkie's label always identifies it as "Golden Sponge Cake," but that gold does not come from a precious metal found in the ground. It comes from a precious liquid found in the ground, sometimes called "black gold." Yes, Red No. 40 and Yellow No. 5 are made from oil, some processed by European companies, some by domestic companies, but most likely from Chinese petroleum refined in the Yellow River Delta, at the edge of the Yellow Sea.

FROM THE YELLOW RIVER TO THE MISSISSIPPI RIVER

Benzene, a colorless, light, flammable oil, is one of the first things to come off crude oil when it is heated in a forty-meter-tall steam cracking tower at China's largest refinery, Sinopec, in the Shengli Oilfield on China's east coast, between Beijing and Shanghai. At night, the refinery looks like a not-so-miniature Manhattan, albeit with colorful pipes instead of streets. This is where both artificial red and yellow begin.

Purple Dye and Perfume

Benzene is the source of the basic materials for food colors and other dyes as well as solvents, gasoline additives, plastics, perfume, and, of course, artificial vanilla. Its main job for colors is to make aniline, a colorless, oily, highly poisonous liquid with an acrid, fishy odor. Getting there involves a major industrial effort. Nitric acid and sulfuric acid are mixed with benzene in a reaction that gives off so much heat that it is considered one of the most dangerous processes in the chemical industry. This yields nitrobenzene, a poisonous, oily liquid that smells like almonds and can be found in pesticides and floor polish. Hydrogenating or exposing it to iron reduces nitrobenzene to form aniline.

Toxic or not, aniline is the backbone of the dye industry. It is the basic chemical from which most dyes are made, including inks, paints, and varnishes. British chemist Sir William H. Perkin created what became the first synthetic dye in 1856 (mauve, if you must know) by accidentally discovering aniline dyes while experimenting with derivatives of coal tar,[14] of which there was plenty in those days, leftover from burning and processing coal into coke for iron-making. He had been trying to make quinine and ended up with a dark goo that, when he attempted to clean it with alcohol, dissolved into a dark purple dye. The textile industry snapped it right up, and Perkin went on to synthesize natural fragrances from it as well, laying the groundwork for all artificial food additives and two robust industries that resulted from his "mistakes." Thanks to him, Hostess can add color and flavor to Twinkies.

Secret Salts and Acids

Shanghai Dyestuffs Research Institute Co., Ltd., the largest synthetic food color producer in China, plays a very important role in creating colors: reacting the aniline with a metal sulfate to create sulfanilic acid (a common metal sulfate is magnesium sulfate, aka Epsom salts).

---

14. Because Perkin extracted the aniline from coal tar, and because for years coal tar was the only source of benzene for dyes, they are still known as "coal tar" dyes despite the fact the most of them are made from oil and natural gas.

Meanwhile, Sinopec refines naphtha and ethylene out of more crude oil and combines them to make naphthalene (a rather unlikely subingredient for a food ingredient, this is the main ingredient in old-fashioned mothballs). Shanghai Dyestuffs reacts this with another acid and plain old table salt to make something called Schaeffer's Salt, the key ingredient in both red and yellow.

At this point, as far as the chemistry goes, the companies clam up. Some hints are available, though. Two acids are essential ingredients: nitrous acid (again) to make red, and tartaric acid for yellow. Synthesized from benzene, tartaric acid was first made from other acids in yet another process developed by the ever-creative Swedish chemist Carl Wilhelm Scheele, who also first isolated oxygen, chlorine, and lactic acid, in 1769.

It seems somehow fitting that Yellow No. 5 can start in the Yellow River Delta, even if the chemical has nothing to do with the river's namesake yellow mud. In any case, once the acids and salts are fully processed, they are dried into gray powders—technically salts—and shipped to plants around the world, probably including this almost spotlessly clean chemical plant near the Mississippi River in St. Louis.

Concentration and Going by the Numbers

The highly polished floors have a slight pink tinge to them. Special shoe covers are required to prevent tracking anything around. Of course, considering what they make here, they'd better keep it clean, or there would be no end to the mess. (It takes thirty-six hours to clean the packaging line when it's time to change color runs.)

Most of the dyes are shipped as powders or granules in boxes or small drums. These dyes are so concentrated that there is no need for larger containers, as even the biggest industrial consumers, like

Twinkies' bakers, use only minuscule, microscopic amounts. A flask of water that has been tinted with just one drop from a solution of one-tenth of 1 percent blue dye, the equivalent of a single drop in an eight-ounce glass of water, sits on a counter in the quality control lab, and it is virtually opaque—that's all it takes. A figure of 50 to 100 ppm (parts per million) is typical for cakes, for example, or only 5 to 10 ppm in drinks such as pink lemonade. That's not a whole lot, which is why colors are usually the last items listed on an ingredient list.

Despite their strength, and how little companies use in a single product, more than 17 million pounds of artificial food coloring are made every year in the United States. (This same concentration means that the security at color plants has been beefed up since 9/11, and it's why I'm not giving too many details about my plant visit here.) Some are shipped as liquids, either pure or mixed with solvents such as water, propylene glycol (the kind of alcohol also mixed with flavors), or glycerin, an oily by-product of vegetable-oil refining (also used to make mono and diglycerides). Glycerin is what you usually find in the little supermarket bottles of food coloring on your kitchen shelf.

Judging color quality is not the least bit subjective, as is evidenced by the high-pressure liquid chromatographs and photospectrometers (which represent colors in nanometer-long wavelengths) found in the quality control lab. Next to the lab is a large corporate-looking conference room that serves as a reminder that all the high-tech stuff is useless if it doesn't please the customers—in this case, the major food companies and, ultimately, the mass-market consumers. A bookcase full of client samples represents a perfect cross-section of an American supermarket and its puddings, cereals, candies, yogurts, and so forth (I am sworn to secrecy as to which ones are here).

It seems logical to ask what the numbers 5 and 40 *really* mean, but, curiously, neither numerous industry experts nor the FDA could say, offhand, when asked. It took some digging to reveal that the numbers signify nothing more than the order in which manufacturers submitted the artificial colors to the FDA for approval (each batch made is certified for compliance, too). Color regulations for artificial colors came into being back in 1906, with the first Food Act. There are a few reasons why there are some apparent gaps: most of the missing numbers are for colors approved only for nonfood use (for drugs or cosmetics, the "D&C" part of the name); some were approved and never used; and some may not have been approved at all. (Some were banned for various safety concerns, including Red No. 2 and Violet No. 1.) So Yellow No. 5 is no better than Red No. 40 despite its lower number—it's probably just older. In any case, we only need three primary colors: red, yellow, and blue. All the rest are just variations on a theme, the rainbow of seven basic colors.

When Natural Is Not

Not everything made at the St. Louis factory is synthetic. Boxes full of seeds of dried fruit pods of the evergreen shrub *Bixa orellana*, named after the historian and botanist Don Francisco de Orellana, who worked for the conquistador Pizarro, arrive at the factory from Peru. Still more come in from Brazil and Kenya. These bloodred seeds yield the popular orange-golden yellow colorant annatto (also known as achiote, rocou, bija, orlean, and the poetic CI Natural Orange 4) once the pigments are extracted with a combination of vegetable oils, alkaline solutions, and heat (and organic solvents for nonfood uses).

The ancient Mayans knew annatto since antiquity, using the concentrated red to represent fire, the sun, and blood. We use it mostly for the much less dramatic task of coloring cheese. Popular in both seed and powder form, it is easily found in grocery stores that cater to Latin Americans, who use it to give a basic golden yellow hue to rice and chicken dishes.

There are twenty-five other natural (or exempt, as in "exempt from certification") colors made at color companies around the world, the most common being: turmeric (a deep yellow from the tuber of a five-foot-tall flowering green plant grown primarily in Cochin, India); anthocyanins (a red/pink/violet from grape skins, red cabbage, elderberries, black currants or other fruit and vegetable juices); titanium dioxide (a white mineral mined from iron ore that is also used in white paint); caramel (brown, from carefully burned sugars, usually corn syrup); and carmine, perhaps the most exotic color due to its rather unusual source.

The fascinating, rich magenta carmine, also known as cochineal, is extracted from the dried body of the female cochineal insect. It takes about seventy thousand insects, which accumulate on the paddles of prickly pear cacti and are simply brushed off and dried, to make a pound of colorant. Large plantations are found in Peru, the primary source, but also in Guatemala and the Canary Islands. When Oaxaca, Mexico, was the center of Mexico's monopoly (until their early eighteenth-century revolution), cochineal exports rivaled silver in value. The output of the Canary Islands is used almost exclusively to color the Italian aperitif Campari, but some is found in common foods, such as Dannon's boysenberry yogurt.

The best thing about natural colors is that they are presumed safe, seeing as they occur naturally in food and plants. On the other hand, natural colors are not necessarily as intense or as easy to incorporate into a recipe, as they are three to five times more expensive than petroleum-derived colors (all that food handling costs something), and, more concerning, they might add some unintended flavor to the recipe. Regardless of the hue, artificial colors do not add flavor—a big advantage.

Still, colors derived from natural sources are often made at the same plants as purely chemical ones, and because they have been processed (or synthesized, in the case of beta-carotene), they are simply no longer considered natural. A label describing these colors can say, "color added," "artificial color added," or actually name the color, but it can't say "natural color." The FDA still classifies them as artificial unless they are coloring the very food they come from, e.g. strawberry juice added to strawberry ice cream.

In any case, while it seems that not one natural color is used in Twinkies, sometimes the label has said "color added," which would make me suspect that annatto, the butter and cheese colorant that is popular with their competitors, is indeed in the mix. But their punctuation indicates otherwise. "Color added" is followed by "(yellow 5 red 40)" which would seem to indicate grammatically that they are the only colors involved. The FDA guidelines are simply not as clear as, say, *The Chicago Manual of Style*.

MAGIC AND PISTACHIOS

Sensient's color service lab in its St. Louis plant is essentially colorless. An enormous, antiseptically clean, brightly lit black, white, and gray space with a dozen stations full of clear glass beakers, gray stainless steel sinks and scales, clear glass cabinetry, and black stone counters, it is also seriously quiet. The white walls are almost devoid of color or art, the exception being some color pictures from its brochures. High-pressure liquid chromatographs, Coulter machines that make microscopic measurements of crystals, spectrometers, and computers are gathered at one end. Cubicles devoid of paper line one wall. This is where scientists concoct the color solutions for name-brand food product clients.

An enthusiastic scientist bounds at high speed from spot to spot, calling out to junior associates for supplies, gathering beakers and tiny spatulas. The atmosphere is charged with anticipation. A pinch of dark brown powder dashed into a beaker of water turns it strawberry red (FD&C Red No. 40); a pinch of dark orange powder turns another beaker of water a cheery lemon yellow (FD&C Yellow No. 5). That the dissolved colors are so much brighter than the powder is just a setup, though. The scientist takes another sample, a light brown blend that looks just like cinnamon, and asks me to guess what color the water will turn ("Um, brown?"). He smiles with glee as the water turns a dark, lush green. "You can't judge a book by its cover," he teases. You sure can't, certainly not here.

Now, on to dry mixes. A dash of the powder, shaken with a few tablespoons of dry sugar, yields nothing but a slight beige tinge. A dash of the same color, in "lake" (water-insoluble pigment) form and shaken with the sugar turns it bright green. Put the same powder—the lake—in water and it sinks to the bottom of the clear beaker as if it were sand. Lakes, which are metallic salts (made from aluminum), color dry mixes in their packaged form (think Country Time® Pink Lemonade mix), packaging materials themselves, and in gums and fats—wherever you need a dry color.

As we leave, I pass another black-white-gray lab area and am jolted by the sight of something brightly colored in the middle of the counter, far from any computer: a huge bowl of red pistachios. Work in progress.

CHAPTER 26

Consider the Twinkie

Finding that Twinkies ingredients may come from as far away as Chinese and Middle Eastern oilfields and involve products from facilities as wide-ranging as steel mills and deep mines may be surprising, especially for such a familiar, small, sweet, everyday item. "All this just for a little cake?" is the obvious question. The answer is yes—because the implications extend far beyond the Twinkie.

THE TWINKIE-INDUSTRIAL COMPLEX

When you consider the Twinkie as a product—which it truly is, in every sense of the term—it's not that hard to fathom its link to the world economy. Twinkies' ingredients are the products of a rural-industrial complex, made from a web of chemicals and raw materials produced by or dependent on nearly every basic industry we know. Where do they come from, my kids wanted to know. They come from an international nexus: the Twinkie Nexus.

Twinkies are obviously connected to food industries such as corn, soybeans, wheat, eggs, and milk, but, in fact, Twinkies ingredients are also manufactured with fourteen of the top twenty chemicals made in the United States, not even including salt (which goes into chlorine) or petroleum. The unlikely food subingredients sulfuric acid, ethylene, lime, and phosphoric acid top the list. The Twinkie Nexus is huge and complex.

That industrial aspect of our food—and Twinkies are but one among tens of thousands of processed foods—would be less troubling if it were easier to still see where it all comes from. There is often no terroir to an ingredient, no one place that it is actually *from*. And between commoditization and competition, most industrial food ingredient suppliers are not easily identified. Most of the vitamins are made in China, essentially placing their manufacture beyond normal scrutiny, and most of the enormous and politically powerful agricultural commodity or global chemical conglomerates simply will not make themselves available. The whole scene is quite opaque. These companies' embrace of science is simply limited by their obedience to the marketplace and governmental policies. One only need recall the recent discovery that partially hydrogenated oils, which were supposed to be better for us than butter, are actually worse, because of trans fats, or that they unrelentingly promote the unnatural use of corn to feed cattle, or that they fully embrace genetic engineering. But we love the results and express this feeling unequivocally with our purchasing power, enthusiastically demanding more protein sources, a wider range of food choices, lower prices, presumably safer and less spoiled food. These are plainly political angles on biology— there are choices to be made—so it is up to us to keep on top of things in the food world.

The fact is that chemicals, especially those in foods, are part of nature. Perhaps a pertinent question is, "When does a chemical become a food?" ("It becomes a food when you decide it is a food," is the tantalizingly vague answer offered by a food scientist with whom I spoke. And what about when you use a food ingredient as a chemical—like the use of cellulose gum in oil well drilling?) It appears to be a matter of perspective. Take flour, for example. Even this most basic, common ingredient seems a product of global technology and commerce when you account for the enriching and bleaching that goes into producing it for Twinkies' use. Parse those words—enriched, bleached—and you learn that flour is mixed with some of the most heavily processed chemicals in the world: vitamins and bleach. It takes a global industrial effort to make enriched flour, to build strong bodies—and to make little snack cakes.

From the Cradle of Civilization to Every Supermarket Shelf

Twinkies' role in history is best understood in the inverse: history's role in shaping the ingredient list. If all of civilization started with the farming of barley (to make beer), then all of the innovations since have led directly from flour and baking to the Twinkie and its emblematic quest for perfection in food.

Probably two of the most fascinating aspects of Twinkies ingredients are that the scientific discoveries in the name of shelf life, taste, texture, and reduced cost are directly rooted in the Industrial Revolution, and that the key inventions of ingredients or processes are tied into historic moments. Especially in the United States after the Civil War, mass supply started to feed mass demand that existed thanks to the arrival of mass communication and transportation systems. The developments are all connected.

Over the years, wars and politics, as key events in history, played key roles in inspiring the development of things like the modern, mechanized flour mill, baking soda, baking powder, artificial colors, artificial flavors, corn syrup, sorbic acid, and polysorbate 60 by forcing manufacturers to find alternative or better sources of subingredients. And these are all ingredients that make the modern Twinkie, as well as all processed food, possible. Late twentieth-century mastery of technology, coupled with the enormous post–World War II consumer demand for convenience and variety as family life became more fractured by demands of the workplace and leisure activities, pushed food scientists and the food companies to even higher levels of creativity that affect almost everything we eat, well beyond a simple snack cake born during the Depression.

This natural evolution led in the early twenty-first century to a highly profitable global processed food market worth $3.2 trillion, one that almost no modern household can do without.

No Cream in the Creme

Shouldn't we be able to admit that we already know that chemicals have always been in our food, and that food is made of chemicals? In fact, food additives—some as old and simple as salt and sugar—keep good food from going bad, and thus prevent food from occasionally killing us. In fact, all food is chemicals and all cooking is chemistry ("Cooking is just science that's tasty," the old saying goes). Remember, the chemicals hydrogen oxide, cellulose, hemicellulose, malic acid, dextrose, fructose, pectin, sucrose, amylacetate, and citric acid are found in nature's perfect food: the apple (in fact, that is the apple's complete ingredient list).

While there is no reason to be paranoid—these additives have been tested and in use for ages—there is reason to be vigilant. That may be what fuels the very negative reaction to genetically modified foods (GM) in Europe, something that is only beginning here. Now the competing consumer trends of natural or organic foods versus traditional convenience foods are coming into sharper focus and voices on both sides are becoming more shrill.

To underscore the confusion around the question of the healthfulness of artificial ingredients, try reflecting on the fact that one of the world's most lethal chemicals, chlorine, and one of the most reactive chemicals, sodium, have an exalted place on every table in the Western world: the salt shaker. Or reduced to the absurd: should the ingredient H_2O scare us because it is often found mixed in with acids and poisons? Shall we sound the alarm? How about those food scientists who manipulate molecules to make new foods? But wait—isn't moving molecules around what you do when you fry an egg or bake a cake or even boil water?

In fact, it's not just the commercial bakers who put unpronounceables in their cakes—you do, too, when you add baking powder, enriched, bleached flour, or even shortening to your homemade confections. "It just ain't plain eggs and butter, pal," as one friendly chef once told me. Examining the labels found on supermarket shelves, it becomes obvious that Twinkies are merely an archetype of almost all modern processed foods; so many others share their ingredients and attempts at immortality on the shelf, ranging from Oreos® (which can last six months) to Freihofer's® 100% Whole Wheat Bread. And contrary to the old joke, Twinkies still won't survive a nuclear war. They're just food. One that lots of us like, and have for a good long time.

All artificial ingredients, like recipes, reflect the balance of various needs (or our perceptions of needs) such as shelf life (long), taste (sweet), texture (fat), convenience (high), price (low), packaging (airtight), nutrition (sound), and legal requirements—and none would exist if there was no profit in it. All are needs generated by our way of life. It seems that we are, indeed, what we eat.

Back when the original Twinkie was low-tech, it was not good for anyone to find a spoiled cake on a shelf. Before getting on a high horse to decry the excessive pressures of capitalism that force food to be so overwhelmingly engineered, we need to remember this: no farmer would bring his or her crops to market without the promise of a reward. Modern food technology is a growth business. On the retail end, packaged food and soft drinks generate close to $400 billion in U.S. sales each year—and their suppliers, whether processors of corn or colors, are large corporations dependent on growth to survive. They fan the flames of consumer demand to maintain the marketplace.

CONSIDER THE TWINKIE

"Good living is an act of intelligence, by which we choose things which have an agreeable taste rather than those which do not," said Jean Anthelme Brillat-Savarin in his seminal 1825 book on gastronomy, *The Physiology of Taste*. Would he have accepted the Twinkie as a culinary achievement?

Pick up a package. The appealing little finger cake just begs to be eaten. It is an appetizing size. Droplets of lush moisture cling teasingly to the inside of the perfectly clear wrapper. Rip it open, feel the softness. Take a bite, not a nibble, and you'll be hit, all at once, with sweetness, stickiness, and a rapidly dissolving texture.

Then comes a second hit of sweetness. Explore the filling with your tongue. Notice the synergy of flavors that build—butter, egg, vanilla—then the creamy finish that lingers, sticky, sweet, and thick. Appreciate the contrast and interplay between the smooth, cool filling and the delicate cake.

Eat enough of 'em, and you'll be able to suss out the bouquet of fresh, Delaware polysorbate 60, and good Georgian cellulose gum; a hint of prime Oklahoman calcium sulfate, or that fine, Midwestern soybean shortening, if not the finest high fructose corn syrup Nebraska has to offer.

Twinkie, deconstructed.

At least now you know what you're eating.

HUMAN RESOURCES

I'd like to thank the dozens of industry professionals who offered time and knowledge despite the press of their daily responsibilities that included little distractions like running billion-dollar plants, traveling the world over, and responding to paying customers. Many of the people listed here responded to my queries as professionals or individuals and not just as corporate representatives, so I am doubly grateful. They all provided a hands-on, real-life perspective for the information that I gathered from the more traditional sources, such as encyclopedias, the Web, industry media, and books. Some of them granted interviews in person, others over the phone, and many responded to numerous questions by e-mail, for which I am especially grateful. A number of them took me on long plant tours and tolerated dozens of follow-up and fact-checking questions, going well beyond the norm of general helpfulness.

Many technical support, sales, or management people helped anonymously as part of their daily toil or just out of professional curiosity and admirable generosity. Despite being unlisted here, they played an essential role in my research over the last several years. I'm sorry I cannot mention them all (and some of them did not wish themselves or their companies to be credited).

Some of the people listed here reviewed the chapters concerning their products and offered corrections, but while that was extremely generous and helpful of them, I remain responsible for any errors that may have managed to creep in.

Sources of general baking, nutrition, food product manufacturing, or scientific information included: Betsy Chotin, Chotin Consulting; Michele C. Fisher, Ph.D., R.D., and Bob Fisher, Ph.D., Food & Nutrition Enterprises, LLC; Jeanne Goldberg, Ph.D., Tufts University Friedman School of Nutrition Science and Policy; Margery Helm, Culinary Delights Catering; Mical Honigfort, United States Food and Drug Administration (FDA); Matthew Jacobson, Operative Cake Company; Jozef Kokini, Ph.D., and William Franke, Ph.D., Rutgers University Center for Advanced Food Technology; Dave Krishock, FNEF Baking Instructor, Grain Science and Industry Department, Kansas State University; Joe Laffin, Southern Signature Foods; Jean C. Lange, M.S., M.P.S., ATR, Pratt Institute; Ronald L. Madl, Ph.D., Director, BIVAP, Grain Science and Industry Department, Kansas State University; Joe Regenstein, Ph.D., Department of Food Science, Cornell University; Laszlo P. Somogyi, Ph.D., Consulting Food Scientist, Teltec, a Division of FIND/SVP; Josh Sosland, Sosland Publishing Company; John Weiser, M.D.; and from the American Institute of Baking, Maureen Olewnick, VP, Stephen L. Sollner, baking instructor, and Tammy Popejoy and Meghan Dowdy, librarians.

✳

The following people were especially generous with time and information in the form of long or repeated interviews and/or tours: Elias Alonso, Keith Krumholz, Dan Murray, and Joseph W. Swink, M.S., Lonza; Greg Anderson, farmer, Nebraska; Edna Anness, East Providence Historical Society; David Astraukas, Twin

Rivers Technologies, Inc.; Charles Baker, Ph.D., and Cheryl Digges, The Sugar Association; James T. Barron, Dan Border, Dennis Grove, and Mark Willis, Morton International; Tim Bebee, Jason Mathews, Michael Foods Egg Products; Maury Belcher, Ag Processing, Inc.; Michael M. Bell and Carlton Windsor, Rayonier; Troy Boutté, Ph.D., Bill Gambel, and Bill Olson, American Ingredients, Inc.; Bill Brady and Eric Johnson, Cargill, Inc.; Derek Budgel, Tembec, Inc.; Denise Broughton, Sondra Dowdell, Chuck LaPorte, Buckeye, Inc.; Kimberlee Burrington, Wisconsin Center for Dairy Research; Mike Cadwell, Firmenich; Sandra Caputo, Hercules, Incorporated/Aqualon; Paul Caulkins, Imperial Sugar; Peter A. Ciullo, sodium bicarbonate writer; Bob Clair, Farbest; Trent L. Clark, Monsanto, Inc.; Maggie Conklin, Charles Bowman and Company; Tim Cottrell and Doug Rector, Kerry Bio-Science; Leon Corzine, corn and soybean farmer, Illinois; Tim Davis, Glenda Thomas, and Jim Wilson, FMC Corporation; Sue Dichter, Dave Hollingshead, Loren Miller, W. Dale Reynolds (retired) and Dennis Socha, United States Gypsum Co.; Gavin Dooley, Daicel Chemical Industries; Joe Ebeling, Mississippi Lime Co.; Karen Endress, Joel Wenk, Alto Dairy; Edward Ettlinger, Peter Ettlinger, and Richard Ettlinger, The Ettlinger Corporation; Susan Feldman, The Salt Institute; Mike Geiger, American Casein; Sharon Gerdes, Dairy Management, Inc.; John Gill, Papettis Hy-Grade Egg Products; Victor Go, BASF; Steve Goewert, The Solae Company; Graham Hall, Bill Riha, Nutrinova, Inc.; Steve Hines, United Sugar; Leonard E. Johnson, Ph.D., DSM Nutritional Products, Inc.; Wanda Jurlina, CP Kelco; Joyce Kilely, Flavor Sciences; Edmund P. Klein, Dow Jones Newswires; Joe Kuterbach, Lyondell Chemical; John LeDonne, Rhodia/Innosphos; M. Stephen Lajoie, Church & Dwight Co., Inc.; Joseph Light, Randy Holme, National Starch; Penny Martin and Harry Meggos, Sensient Colors, Inc.; Nancy McDonald, M&M Consulting; Pam Meeks, Clabber Girl Corporation; Don Morton, Maize Associates; Matt Nielsen,

Nielsen-Massey Vanillas; J. Scott Peterson, Crown Technology; Peter Ranum, Ceres Nutrition; Steve Schorn, Research Products Company; Fred Schubert, Friends Seminary; Kevin Shoemaker, Purac, Inc.; Hugh Smith, Prestige Proteins; Terry Smith, PPG Chloralkali Chemicals; Bob Smolenowski, Borregaard; Dr. L. Jay Stoel, Reilly Industries, Inc.; Tom Suber, U.S. Dairy Export Council; Doug Sweet, Federated Mills; Florian Ward, Ph.D., VP of R&D, Tic Gums, Inc.; John S. White, Ph.D., White Technical Research; and Dick Wilkinson, Martin Gas. Please forgive me if I have omitted anyone.

✳

Several editorial assistants helped me in various ways and at different times over two years, for either research or manuscript preparation, including Liz Dobricki, Tim Guetterman, Amelie Hayte, Jessica Silver-Greenberg, Rachel Tubman, Mel Wathen, Zhang Yifei (in China), and especially Leslie Kaufmann and Sara Watson. Thanks to all of you for working hard and odd hours to accommodate me.

INDEX

Acacia gum, 123
Acetaldehyde, 36
Acetic acid, 154, 210, 241
Acetone, 41, 94
Acetylene, 35–36, 210
Acid hydrolysis, 1, 59, 663
Adhesives, 67, 96, 97, 172, 227, 229, 235
Ag Processing Inc., 90, 92, 103
Ahmann, Steve, 158
Alkali Act, 148
Alkali chemical lye, 22
All in the Family (television show), 5
Allied Custom Gypsum, 232
Alonso, Elias, 35
Alpha amylase, 61, 63
Alto Dairy Cooperative, 129
American Cookery (Simmons), 135
American Ingredients, 41, 181–185, 217, 221–223

American Sugar Refining Inc., 51*n*
Amines, 30, 36
Amino acids, 41, 59, 65, 106, 109, 154, 227
Amish farms, 14
Ammonia, 30, 35, 36, 103
Ammonium carbonate, 37
Ammonium nitrate, 37
Amylacetate, 260
Anaheim, California, 206
Anderson, Greg, 88, 89
Anderson, Richard, 70
Anemia, 40
Aniline, 250, 251
Animal feed, 57, 59, 81, 88, 109, 111, 258
Annatto, 253–255
Anthocyanins, 254
Antibiotics, 59, 65
Apopka, Florida, 200

Archer Daniels Midland (ADM), 16, 55, 56, 80, 90, 94, 119

Arctic National Wildlife Refuge, 175

Argo, 76

Arm & Hammer Baking Soda, 143, 149

Arrowroot starch, 59

Arsenic, 157

Artificial butter, 210–213

Artificial colors (*see* Food coloring)

Artificial vanilla, 33, 197, 202, 205–210, 212, 213, 250

Ashbya gossypii fungus, 38

Aspartame, 40

Aspirin, 207, 241

Astraukas, Dave, 193

Atlas Powder Company, 188–189, 194

B vitamins, 31, 32, 36

Bacillus subtilis, 38

Backward integration, 36

Bakelite, 207

Baking powder, 9, 75, 76, 84, 133, 134, 137–139, 153, 154, 162, 164, 166, 167, 259

Baking process, 46–47, 84

Baking soda, 133, 134, 136, 137, 139, 141–152, 153, 163, 259

Banana, 201

BASF, 31, 37, 211

Baton Rouge, Louisiana, 205, 207

Beauharnois, Canada, 22

Beaumont, Texas, 22

Bebee, Tim, 113

Beef fat, 91, 92, 100, 101*n*, 197

Beer, 64, 66, 134, 219–221, 235

Belcher, Maury, 92

Bell, Don, 117

Ben & Jerry's ice cream, 107

Benzene, 206–208, 249–250

Beriberi, 29, 30, 37

Beta-carotene, 255

Better'n Eggs, 216

Betty Crocker Whipped Vanilla Frosting, 197

Biotechnology, 30

Birth defects, 30, 40

Blair, Nebraska, 57, 58, 74, 217–218

Bleach
  flour, 9, 20, 21–28
  household, 21, 24

Blood sugar, 60, 66

Borden, 227

Borden, Gail, Jr., 227

Boutté, Troy, 181, 184, 222, 223

Boyle, Jimmy, 13–14, 16

Brand, Henning, 156–157

Bread, 8, 15, 66, 73, 95, 134, 135, 216, 234

Breyers Carb Smart Ice Cream Bars, 228

Brillat-Savarin, Jean Anthelme, 262

Brine, 25

British gums, 80

Brooklyn, New York, 52

Brown rice, 30, 37

Browning, 47–48, 64, 65–68, 106, 126

Bruno, Don, 41, 42

Butane, 211

Butter, 99, 100, 102, 126, 179, 189, 197, 200, 201, 210, 211, 248
    artificial, 210–213
Butyric acid, 41, 212

Cadwell, Mike, 206–207
Calcium, 126, 133, 160, 165
Calcium carbonate, 232
Calcium caseinate, 85, 225–229
Calcium fluorapatite, 156
Calcium hydroxide (*see* Lime)
Calcium lactate, 219–220
Calcium lime, 161
Calcium oxide, 162, 167
Calcium sorbate, 241
Calcium sulfate, 9, 10, 84, 85, 138, 160–161, 220, 229, 231–238, 263
Candida yeasts, 38
Candies, 66, 76, 193
Candles, 98, 217*n*
Cane molasses, 41
Cane sugar industry, 45*n*
Canola oil, 38, 91–92, 99, 181, 182, 197
Caramel, 254
Carbohydrates, 38, 60
Carbolic acid, 207
Carbon, 37
Carbon atoms, 100
Carbon dioxide, 46, 53, 147, 151, 242
Carbon monoxide, 6, 34, 212, 240, 241
Carbonated beverages, 66
Cardboard, 73, 79
Cargill, 16, 57–59, 61, 67–68, 70, 72, 74, 217–218
Carmine, 254

Carpenter, David, 156
Casein, 225, 226
Caseinates, 10, 225–229
Catechol, 202, 207
Caustic soda (*see* Sodium hydroxide)
Celanese, 243
Cellulose, 260
Cellulose gum, 9, 85, 115–123, 189, 259, 262–263
Center for Science in the Public Interest (CSPI), 242
Cheese, 123, 125, 127, 129, 131, 171, 179, 225, 253
Cheetos, 218
Chemical industry, 7–8, 26, 32–33
Chemical Weapons Convention, 23
Chewing gum, 95, 128, 191
Chicago, Illinois, 139, 161, 164–165
Chickens, 38, 108–110
Chlor/alkali industry, 21–22, 172, 217, 261
Chlorine, 9, 21–28, 78, 172, 173, 210, 251, 258
Chlorine gas, 23–24, 26, 28
Chocolate, 95, 171
Cholesterol, 100
Church, Austin, 148–149
Church, James, 149
Citric acid, 59, 65, 154, 260
Citrus extract, 30
Citrus fruits, 40
Clabber Girl, 138, 139
Clinton, Iowa, 55
Clinton Corn Processing Company, 56

Clove oil, 206
Coal tar, 37, 206, 250
Coca-Cola, 8, 69, 71, 154
Cochineal, 254
Coconut oil, 182, 197
Cod liver oil, 38
Coffee-mate, 228
Coke, 157, 250
Cold Stone Creamery, 180
Colonization, 50
Coloring (*see* Food coloring)
Columbus, Christopher, 50
Con-Agra, 16
Coniferin, 205
Continental Bakeries, 7
Corn, 9, 56–58, 70, 74–76, 88–90,
    109, 190, 223, 258
Corn: Part of a Healthy Diet (Corn
    Refiners Association), 68
Corn chips, 81
Corn flour, 25, 73, 80–81, 85
Corn oil, 181, 242
Corn Refiners Association, 68
Corn sweetener industry, 45*n*
Corn sweeteners, 54, 55–63
Corn syrup, 45, 46, 58–65, 68, 80,
    112, 121, 129, 191, 194, 209,
    218, 219, 260
Cornflakes, 81
Cornmeal, 36, 81
Cornstarch, 41, 59, 60, 62, 63, 72,
    73–81, 85, 138, 235
Corriher, Shirley O., 94
Corzine, Leon, 56
Cosettes, 53
Cosmetics, 67, 75, 96, 122, 128,
    172, 182, 191–193, 197, 209,
    217*n*
Cotton, 115, 116, 118, 119, 123

Cottonseed oil, 91, 99, 181, 182
Council Bluffs, Iowa, 90
Crabtree & Evelyn, 192
Cream, 102, 121, 126, 127, 180, 189
Crisco, 90, 97, 99–101, 180–181
Crotanaldehyde, 240, 241
Crown Technology, 34
Crude oil, 32
Cumene, 207
Cunningham, Mary Lou, 191

Daicel Chemical Industries, 240
Dairy Fresh Non-Dairy Creamer,
    99
Davis, Tim, 142, 145, 146
Davy, Sir Humphry, 22
Decatur, Illinois, 90
Deep tank technology, 33–34
Delmarva area, 13–14
Deltadodecalactone, 212
Denk, Joel, 130, 131
Denture adhesives, 122
Detergents, 62, 164
Devil Cremes, 6
Dewar, James, 7
Dextrin, 64, 75, 77, 79
Dextrose, 61, 62, 64, 65–67, 71,
    178, 191, 218, 219, 260
Diabetes, 68–70
Diacetyl, 202, 210–212
Diesel fuel, 81, 97, 183
Diglycerides, 3, 85, 95, 99,
    179–185, 188, 190, 193, 221
Diketene, 240, 241
DingDongs, 6
Directional drilling, 175
DNA, 154
Domino Sugar, 51, 52
Domino Superfine, 47

Donut Pyro, 166
Doonesbury comic strip, 4–5
Doritos, 127
Doritos Nacho Cheese, 66
Dove Beautifully Clean
    Shampoo, 193
Dow Chemical, 116, 183, 195, 209
Dried eggs, 112–114
Dried milk, 126, 226, 227
Dry milling, 80–81
DSM, 31
Duncan Hines Creamy
    Homestyle Cream Cheese
    Frosting, 190
DuPont, 32, 103, 188
Durum, 15
Dwight, John, 148–149
Dye industry, 250

Eagle Brand Sweetened
    Condensed Milk, 48
Easy Cheese, 127
Edamame, 89
Edy's Grand Light Rich &
    Creamy Vanilla ice cream,
    180
Egg whites, 106, 107, 111, 228
Egg yolks, 94, 95, 106, 107, 111,
    180, 189, 216, 223
Eggs, 8, 10, 104, 105–114, 126,
    134, 226, 258
Eijkman, Christiaan, 37
Electricity, 22, 24, 25
Elizabeth, New Jersey, 105, 107,
    112, 113
Elmer's glue, 227
Enoch Valley Mine, Idaho,
    155–156
Enriched flour, 8, 29–44

Entenmann's cakes, 107
Enzymes, 60–65, 129, 244
Equistar, 195, 209
Eskimo Pie Ice Cream Bars, 197
Ethane, 194, 195, 240
Ethanol, 38, 65, 81
Ethyl acetate, 202
Ethyl alcohol, 65
Ethyl cellulose, 116
Ethyl maltol, 209
Ethyl vanillin, 202
Ethylene, 35–36, 195, 251, 258
Ethylene glycol, 209
Ethylene oxide, 194–196, 240
Evans, Oliver, 136
Everglades Agricultural Area, 49
Explosives, 48, 81, 96, 154,
    188–189, 195
ExxonMobil, 151, 195

Famous Amos cookies, 107
Faraday, Michael, 24
Farmers, 13–14, 56
Fermentation, 30, 32, 39, 40,
    58–59, 64, 66, 203, 219, 244
Ferric oxide, 34
Ferrous sulfate, 33–34, 42, 43
Fertilizers, 154, 156
Fiberglass, 163
Firmenich Inc., 204, 206
Fish, 38
Flavor Sciences Inc., 199, 200
Flavors, 199–213
Fleur de sel, 173
Florida Crystals Corporation, 51
Flour, 10, 45, 85, 136, 172, 259
    bleached, 9, 20, 21–28
    enriched, 8, 29–44
    wheat, 13–20

FMC Corporation, 139, 142–147, 150–152, 163–164, 217
Folate, 40–41
Folic acid, 30, 40–43
Food and Drug Administration (FDA), 29, 40, 66, 172, 205, 241, 252–253, 255
Food coloring, 10, 25, 171, 183, 245, 247–256, 260
Forbes magazine, 57
Formaldehyde, 206, 207
Fractionation units, 71
Franklin, Benjamin, 233
Freeport, Texas, 183
Freihofer's 100% Whole Wheat Bread, 261
Frozen eggs, 112, 113
Fructose, 69–71, 260
Fudgsicles, 127
Funk, Casimir, 30
Furfural, 209

Geismar, Louisiana, 160
Gelatinization, 47
Generally recognized as safe (GRAS), 172, 241
Genetic engineering, 30, 258
Genetically modified (GM) seeds, 56n, 260
Geneva Convention, 24
Gill, John, 108
Glass, 142, 143, 147, 163
Glop, 94
Glucose, 38, 60, 62, 64–67, 69
Glucose amylase, 62
Glucose isomerase, 62, 71
Glue, 79–80
Glutamate, 65
Glutamic acid, 41

Gluten, 15, 16, 27, 59, 85, 102
Glycerin, 182–183, 188, 189, 193, 209, 252
Glycerol, 183
Glyoxylic acid, 208
Gobley, Maurice, 94
Good Humor ice cream bars, 127
Grand Saline, Texas, 174
Grandview, Missouri, 181, 183, 217, 221
Great Depression, 6–7
Green River, Wyoming, 139, 142, 147, 163–164, 217
Grits, 81
Grove, Dennis, 176
Guaiacol, 207–209
Guaifenesin, 207
Guangji Pharmaceutical Company, 39
Guar gum, 123
Gum arabic, 123
Gypsum (*see* Calcium sulfate)

Harvard University, 136–137
Hay, 16
Heliotropine, 202, 209
Hellmann's mayonnaise, 107
Helms, Allen, 118
Hemicellulose, 118, 260
Herbicides, 87, 160
Hercules Incorporated, 120, 189
Hexane, 91–93
High fructose corn syrup (HFCS), 1, 2, 4, 45, 56, 58, 62, 65, 67–72, 263
Hines, Steve, 53
Hippocrates, 131
Ho Hos, 6
Hoffman, A. W., 242

Hoffman-La Roche, 31
Hollingshead, Dave, 236
Homegrown food, 2
Homogenization, 112
Honey, 64
Horsford, Eben Norton, 137–138
Hostess, 5, 7, 34, 66, 83, 106, 120–121, 127, 201
Household bleach, 21, 24
Hunt's Snack Pack Vanilla Pudding, 216
Hydrochloric acid (HC1), $25n$, 27, 35, 38, 60, 63, 78, 79, 103, 148, 164, 210, 211, 229
Hydrogen, 25, 34, 193, 212, 250
Hydrogen atoms, 100
Hydrogen oxide, 260
Hydrogen peroxide, 37
Hydrogenation, 97–101

I Can't Believe It's Not Butter, 180
Ice cream, 8, 64, 66, 95, 107, 116, 122, 127, 180, 197, 210, 228, 248
IG Farben, 116
Indianapolis, Indiana, 7, 75, 200
Industrial espionage, 58
Infant formula, 104, 127
Innophos, 139, 160, 161, 164–168
Insulin, 70
International Flavors and Fragrances (IFF), 201
International Food Information Council (IFIC), 69
Iodine, 178
Iron, 9, 32, 34
Iron deficiency anemia, 29
Iron ore, 33
Iron salt, 34

Iron sulfate, 34
Isomerization, 71

Jams, 66, 122, 154
Jean Naté Hydrating Body Lotion, 197
Jefferson, Thomas, 204
Jell-O Pudding Snacks, 216
Jellies, 66, 122, 154
Johnson, Eric D., 58, 61, 72

Karo Light corn syrup, 63
Ken's Steak House Creamy Italian Dressing, 190
Ketchup, 41
Ketene, 241
Kiley, Joyce, 199–201
Kingsford, Thomas, 75
Kingsford's Starch, 75–76
Kirchoff, G. S. C., 59–60
KLK (Kuala Lumpur Kepong Berhad), 192
Knorr Instant Hollandaise Sauce Mix, 79
Kosher food, 96, $101n$, 182, 183, 237
Kraft
  American cheese, 127
  Calumet Double-Acting Baking Powder, 235
  Cheez Whiz, 127
  Cool Whip, 102, 190
  Free French Style Fat-Free Dressing, 65
  Jet-Puffed Marshmallows, 78
  Sure-Jell Premium Fruit Pectin for Homemade Jams & Jellies, 66
Kreme Filled Krimpets, 6

Krishock, Dave, 79
Kunz, Gray, 3, 179

Lactic acid, 33, 51, 65, 129,
    218–222, 244, 251
Lactones, 212
Lactose, 126, 127, 129, 130
Lafayette, Indiana, 7
Lake Charles, Louisiana, 22
Lard, 97n, 99, 197
Lauric acid, 197
Laxatives, 122
Leavenings, 46, 47, 106, 132,
    133–139
Leblanc, Nicolas, 148
Lecithin, 85, 88, 89, 91, 93–97,
    103, 180, 190
Lemon juice, 136
Lespinasse restaurant, 3
Lignin, 118, 206
Lime, 51, 53, 63, 103, 133, 161, 162,
    164, 172, 219, 229, 233, 258
Limestone, 133, 153, 161, 167,
    172, 232
Linolenic soybeans, 101
Liquid nitrogen, 221
Liquid petroleum gas, 35
Liquid starch, 59, 63, 74
Liquid sugar, 47, 54
Lister, Sir Joseph, 207
Little Debbie, 5, 150
    Golden Cremes, 6
Liver, 30, 38, 40
Lonza Ltd., 35
Louis XVI, King of France, 148
Low-fat foods, 78–79
Lye, 78, 80, 103, 120, 164, 172,
    210, 217, 229
Lysine, 106, 109

Magnesium sulfate, 250
Maillard reactions, 65, 68, 106
Malic acid, 260
Maltodextrin, 64
Maltol, 202
Mannitol, 189
Margarine, 94, 180, 192
Marggraf, Andreas, 53
Marion, Arkansas, 118
Marmite, 40
Marshmallow Fluff, 64
McCormick and Company, 200,
    201, 204
    Au Jus Gravy Mix, 122
McDonald, Nancy, 200, 201
McElvaney, Kevin, 52, 54
Meth production, 159
Methane, 5, 240
Methanol, 38, 240–241
Methyl esters, 182–183, 207
Methyl ethyl ketone (MEK), 211
Michael Foods, 105, 113
Milk, 38, 123, 126–132, 167, 179,
    218–219, 223, 225–227, 229,
    258
Millet seeds, 38
Mississippi Lime Company, 161,
    219
M&M Consulting and
    Laboratory, 200
Modified cornstarch, 75, 78–79
Moisture control, 10, 48, 49, 67,
    77, 78, 81
Molasses, 51, 52, 54, 94
Monocalcium phosphate (MCP),
    134, 137, 139, 153, 161,
    165–167, 219
Monoglycerides, 3, 85, 95, 99,
    179–185, 188, 190, 193, 221

Monosodium glutamate (MSG), 41, 65
Monsanto, 56n, 155, 157–160
  Roundup, 160
  Roundup Ready seeds, 87
Morder, Dan, 173
Morton, 169–171, 173–178
Mountain ash tree (Sorbus aucuparia), 242–243
Mountain Fuel Supply, 142
Mrs. Freshley's Creme Cakes, 45
Myths surrounding Twinkies, 4, 6, 47

Nantong Acetic Acid Chemical Company, 240
Naphtha, 35, 251
Naphthalene, 251
Napoleon, 60, 72
Nashville, Tennessee, 160
National Starch, 74, 75
Natural gas, 78, 202–203, 206, 209, 240
Naval jelly, 154
Neutrogena
  Norwegian Formula Hand Cream, 193
  Oil-Free Acne Wash, 197
New Castle, Delaware, 188, 191, 194
New Coke, 204
Newman Grove, Nebraska, 88
Niacin, 35–36, 43
Niagara Falls, New York, 21, 22
Nielsen, Matt, 204, 205
Nielsen-Massey Vanillas, 204
Night-blindness, 30
Nitric acid, 36, 37, 250, 251
Nitrobenzene, 250

Nitrogen, 20, 35–36, 172, 211, 220
Nitroglycerin, 182, 188
Niutang Chemical Inc., 40
Nutraceuticals, 127
Nutrament energy and fitness drink, 228
Nutrinova (Hoechst AG), 240, 242, 243
Nutrition bars, 127
Nutrition Facts labels, 101

Obesity, 68–70
Occidental Petroleum Corporation, 22
Ocean Spray Ruby Red Grapefruit Juice, 248
Oil palms, 190, 192
Olay Moisturinse Shower Body Lotion, 197
Oleic acid, 197
Olive oil, 180, 182, 197, 242
Olivio, 180
Olsen, Bill, 41, 42
Oreos, 261
Oscar Mayer Turkey Bologna, 76
Oswego, New York, 75
Oxidation, 26, 37
OxyChem, 22, 23
Oxygen, 35, 166, 172, 195, 212, 221, 251

Paint, 96, 97, 209, 226
Palladium, 240
Palm kernel oil, 92, 182, 183, 192
Palm oil, 91, 92, 99, 181–183, 192–194
Palm trees, 216
PAM cooking spray, 96

Paper, 73, 117–119, 164, 172, 206
Papetti's Hygrade Egg products, 105, 107, 108, 110–113
Papyrus, 75
Paraffin, 42, 98
Partially hydrogenated vegetable shortening, 94, 96–100, 102, 258
Pasteur, Louis, 138
Pasteurization, 112
Peanut butter, 95, 102, 180
Pearlash, 135, 136, 147
Pebble quicklime, 162
Pectin, 66, 122, 260
Pellagra, 29, 36
Penicillin, 59, 65
Peoria, Illinois, 80
Periodic table, 24
Perkin, Sir William H., 250
Pesticides, 78
Peterson, J. Scott, 34
Petroleum, 9, 33, 35, 40, 78, 172, 183, 190, 206, 207, 209, 211, 240, 249, 258
Pharmaceuticals, 66, 67, 78, 164, 191, 207, 209, 235
Phenol, 202, 207
Phosphates, 9, 133, 153–168, 172, 232
Phosphoric acid, 8–9, 33, 78, 137, 153–155, 158, 160, 164–166, 258
Phosphorus, 133, 153–159, 220
Phosphorus oxychloride, 78
Physiology of Taste, The (Brillat-Savarin), 262
Pickle liquor, 33
Pickling process, 33
Pine Bluff, Arkansas, 119

Pine needle extract, 30
Pine trees, 117
Pizza, 15, 16, 47, 73
Planters Cotton Oil Mill, 119
Plaque, 100
Plaster, 9, 160, 231, 233–234, 236, 237
Plastic, 65, 96, 128, 172, 194, 195, 207, 217n, 226
Platinum, 240
Pockle (phosphorus, oxygen, chloride [P-O-C]), 78
Point of origin, 2
Pollution, 31, 148, 157–158
Polyethylene, 35
Polysorbate 20, 196–197
Polysorbate 60, 1, 3, 4, 9, 65, 85, 95, 99, 121, 180, 185, 187–197, 216, 240, 260, 262
Polysorbate 80, 196–197
Polyurethane foam, 48
Potassium bicarbonate, 135
Potassium carbonate, 147
Potassium hydroxide, 22, 241
Potassium iodide, 177
Potassium sorbate, 241
Potatoes, 74
Pound cakes, 27
PPG Industries, 22, 23
Pregelatinized starch, 77
Preservatives, 48, 170, 171, 239–245
Procter & Gamble, 99, 182
Propylene gas, 183, 207, 210
Propylene glycol, 209–210, 212, 252
Propylene oxide, 78, 210
Protein, 10, 15, 16, 26, 27, 47, 103, 106, 126, 127, 129

Pteroic acid, 41
Pteroyl-L-glutamic acid, 41
Purac, 218, 219
PVC (polyvinylchloride), 26

Questar, 142
Quicklime, 162
Quincy, Massachusetts, 192–193, 217

Raw food, 2
Raw sugar, 51, 52
Red No. 40, 3, 9, 85, 247–249, 251–253, 255, 256
Reduced iron, 34–35
Refined sugar, 52–54
Refractometer, 72
Rennet, 129, 229
Rhodia, 32, 201, 205
Riboflavin, 38–39, 42, 43
Rice, 39, 74
Riha, Bill, 242
Rillieux, Norbert, 51
Ring dryer, 75
Ronzoni pasta, 107
Rose hips, 3
Rumford Baking Powder, 138, 139
Rust, 34

Sabatier, Paul, 99
Sackett, Augustine, 234
St. Joseph, Missouri, 90
St. Louis, Missouri, 103
Ste. Genevieve, Missouri, 161
Sal soda, 147, 163
Salad dressings, 8, 64–65, 76, 78, 122, 127, 190
Salaratus, 148–149

Salt, 22, 24, 25, 51, 85, 112, 121, 168, 169–178, 210, 213, 219, 232, 258, 260, 261
Saltpeter, 48
Saturated fats, 100, 101, 181
Schaeffer's Salt, 251
Scheele, Carl Wilhelm, 22, 182, 218–219, 251
Scurvy, 30
Sea salt, 148, 173
Sensient Colors Inc., 247–248, 255
Sensient Technologies, 200
Serving sizes, 69
Sesame seeds, 167
Shanghai Dyestuffs Research Institute Company, Ltd., 250, 251
Sheetrock, 232, 234
Shelf life, 7, 8, 10, 46, 48, 81, 95, 106–107, 120–121, 126, 134, 139, 180, 216, 219, 239
Shellac, 128
Shoemaker, Kevin, 218
Shortening, 90–93, 97n, 97–99, 102, 121, 193
Silica, 157, 163, 233
Silver Springs, New York, 169, 171, 173–176
Simmons, Amelia, 135
Sinopec, 249, 251
Slim-Fast Optima, 121, 228
Smith, Terry, 23, 24
Smuckers Reduced Fat Natural Style Peanut Butter, 64
Soap, 142, 143, 147, 164, 182, 193, 197, 222
Soda ash, 142–143, 146–158, 162–165, 216–217, 223

Soda Springs, Idaho, 153, 155–157

Sodium, 24, 25, 41, 173, 216–217, 261

Sodium acid phosphate, 137

Sodium acid pyrophosphate (SAPP), 134, 139, 143, 153, 164, 165, 216

Sodium aluminum sulfate, 134

Sodium bicarbonate (*see* Baking soda)

Sodium carbonate, 51, 142, 147, 150–153, 161–163, 166, 167, 216, 222

Sodium carboxymethyl-cellulose (CMC), 120, 122

Sodium caseinate, 25, 85, 223, 225–229

Sodium chloride (NaC1), 24

Sodium ferrocyanide, 178

Sodium hydroxide, 22, 24, 25, 63, 80, 97, 172, 217, 229, 247

Sodium methoxide, 217

Sodium monochloroacetate, 120

Sodium nitrite, 247

Sodium sesquicarbonate, 142, 150

Sodium silicoaluminate, 177

Sodium stearate, 222

Sodium stearoyl lactylate, 8, 25, 65, 85, 99, 142, 164, 180, 190, 215–223

Soft drinks, 59, 68, 69, 71–72

Solae Company, 103

Solution mining, 169, 175–176

Solvay process, 149

Sorbic acid (trans trans 2, 4-hexadienoic acid), 10, 85, 107, 191, 239–245, 260

Sorbin, 243

Sorbit, 243

Sorbitan monostearate (SMS), 194, 196

Sorbitol, 65, 99, 191, 243

Sourdough, 135

South Beach Diet, 60

Southard, Oklahoma, 232, 236–237

Soy flour, 91, 93

Soy grits, 93

Soy protein isolate, 25, 85, 88, 89, 91, 93, 103–104

Soybean oil, 25, 38, 94, 98–99, 101, 180, 181, 182, 191, 197, 242

Soybeans, 8, 9, 39, 57, 85, 87–104, 109, 128, 167, 216, 258, 263

Spanish barilla, 147–148

Sparks, Maryland, 200

Spent bee grain, 38

SPI Polyols, 191

Spinach, 40

Sponge cake, 27, 47, 77, 106, 134, 171

Sports drinks, 8, 127

Starbucks
  Frappuccino, 122
  Low Fat Latte ice cream, 122

Starch, 40–41, 61, 74–81

Stearic acid, 22, 99, 182, 191–192, 217, 222

Steel pickling, 33

Steep water, 58

Straw, 16

Sucrose, 46, 49, 64, 68, 69, 71, 260

Sugar, 8, 10, 11, 27, 44, 45–54, 60, 64, 66, 68, 70, 121, 189, 260

Sugar beets, 49, 53, 60

Sugar Trust, 52

Sugarcane, 49–51, 53, 60
Sulfanilic acid, 250
Sulfate, 32
Sulfur, 32–33
Sulfur dioxide, 33, 58, 164
Sulfuric acid, 33–34, 60, 78, 137, 148, 160, 165, 172, 206, 209, 220, 258
Sunflower oil, 91, 101, 181
Surfactant, 96
Suzy Q's, 6
Swiss Miss Hot Cocoa Mix, 122
Sydney, Iowa, 56

Table sugar (*see* Sucrose)
Tallow, 92, 192, 197
Tapioca starch, 41, 74
Tartaric acid, 136, 251
Tate & Lyle, 74
Terre Haute, Indiana, 138
Texas City, Texas, 207
Thiamine, 37, 43
Thiamine hydrochloride, 38
Thiamine mononitrate, 37–38, 42
Thinned starches, 79
Thomas, Glenda, 150, 152
Thompson, Benjamin, 137
Tianjin Zhongjin Pharmaceutical Company, 37
Titanium dioxide, 254
Tobacco, 67
Tofu, 39, 93, 103, 234
Tollhouse Mint Brownie Bars, 127
Toothpaste, 116, 122, 128, 191
Tortillas, 80, 81
Trans fats, 6n, 91, 101, 102, 258
Trees, 115–118, 123, 242–243
Tribasic phosphate, 103

Triglycerides, 70, 179–180, 182, 192
Triscuits, 179
Trona, 133, 142–147, 149–150, 163–164
Trudeau, G. B., 5
Tryptophan, 36
Tums, 161
Turmeric, 254
Twin Rivers Technologies, 192–193, 217
"Twinkie defense," 5

UK Patent Office, 26
Union Pacific Railroad, 163
Union Sugar Company, 60–61
Uniqema, 188, 191, 194
United States Gypsum (USG), 232, 236
United Sugar, 53
University of Iowa, 101
Unsaturated fats, 100
Uranium, 160
Urine, 156–157

Vanadium, 158
Vanadium oxide, 211
Vanilla, 200–205, 208
    artificial, 33, 197, 202, 205–210, 212, 213, 250
Vanillin (4-hydroxy-3-methoxybenzaldehyde), 202, 205–210, 250
Vaseline Intensive Care Dry Skin Lotion, 217n
Vegetable oil, 25, 93, 94, 97, 181
Veggie Slices Cheese Alternative American Flavor Organic, 228

Velveeta cheese sauces, 127
Vinegar, 136
Vitamin B1, 35–36
Vitamin B2, 38–39, 42, 43
Vitamin B3, 35–36, 43
Vitamin B9, 30, 40–41, 40–43
Vitamin C, 3, 65
Vitamins, 20, 28, 29–44, 64, 258
Vulcan Spice Mills, 149

Wakefield, Nebraska, 113
Walsh, Kelly, 248
Wanaque Reservoir, New Jersey, 83
Washing soda, 147, 163, 164
Water, 45, 47, 81, 83–85, 93, 121, 127, 210
Watt, James, 136
Waukegan, Illinois, 204
Waupun, Wisconsin, 128
Waxy maize or corn, 74
Wayne, New Jersey, 52, 83
Western Phosphate Field, 156
Wheat, 8, 13–20, 74, 258
Wheat gluten, 15

Wheat starch, 75
Whey, 10, 51, 85, 125–132, 225–227, 229
Whey protein concentrate, 126, 127
White, Dan, 5
Wills, Lucy, 40
Wise
  Cheez Doodles, 76
  Sour Cream and Onion Potato Chips, 127
Wish-Bone Fat Free Chunky Blue Cheese salad dressing, 122
Wonder Bread, 7, 216, 235
World War I, 23, 60
World War II, 8, 60

Xanthan gum, 65, 123

Yeast, 38, 64, 66, 133–135, 211
Yellow #2 dent field corn, 74
Yellow No. 5, 85, 247, 249, 251–253, 255, 256
Yellow prussiate of soda, 178
Yogurt, 126, 129, 132